Earth Dragon Canon

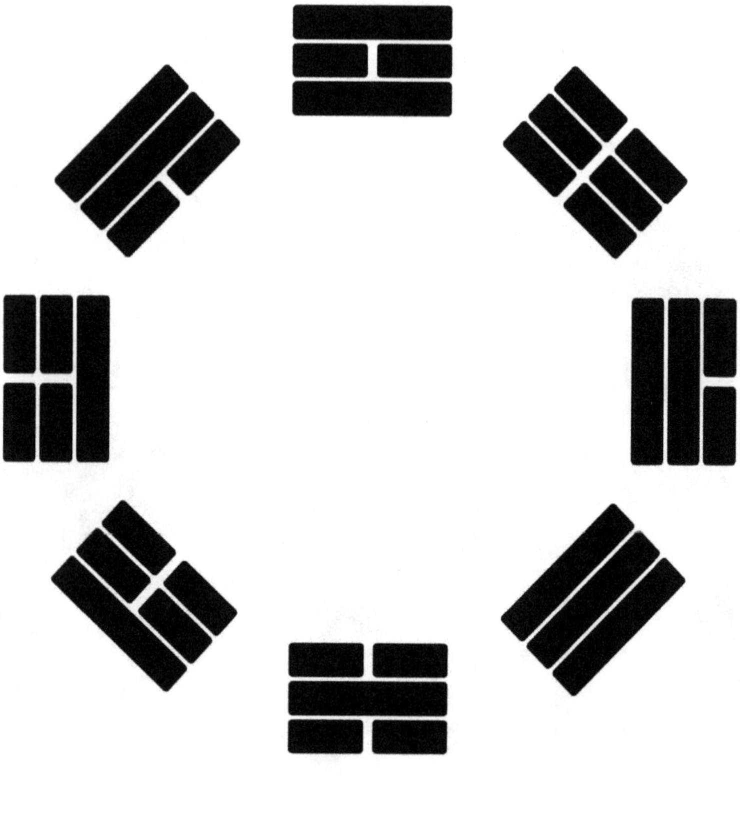

Walking, Martial Arts, and Self Evolution

Published by: The Walking Circle LLC
312 S. Martinson
Wichita Kansas, 67213
http://www.thewalkingcircle.com

First Edition, 2009

Second Edition, 2010

ISBN-13: 9780981967523

ISBN-10: 0981967523

Book and Cover Design: Troy Williams

The authors and publishers of this material are not responsible in any manner for any injury which may occur through following the instructions in this material. The activities, physical or otherwise, described in this material may be too strenuous or dangerous for some people, and readers should consult a physician before engaging in them.

DEDICATION

For Gianna,

Who allowed the dreamer to manifest the dream.

ACKNOWLEDGMENTS

Books are arguments (usually) made by the author with himself. I would like to thank the members of TheWalkingCircle.com who joined this author in his argument with their valuable input: Keith Ahlstrom, K. B., Don Gold, J.P. Hayes, Danny Hess, Bill Kobbs, and Ron Lambert.

TABLE OF CONTENTS

LANGUAGE BARRIER

The Pinyin system is the accepted standard for the romanization of Chinese characters. Pinyin means *spell sound* and is used to teach the standard pronunciation of Mandarin Chinese. It is also the standard system for entering Chinese characters on computers. Because of this standardization it is the method used in this book.

You can be confident that if you pronounce the words as they are written in this book you are close to the actual Chinese pronunciation. I am not a Chinese language speaker, and I do not get these pronunciations correct each time either. The following chart helps me with some tricky characters:

LETTER	PRONUNCIATION	LETTER	PRONUNCIATION
b	**b**ay or s**p**it	p	**p**ay
j	**j**eep or a**j**ar	q	**ch**eer
d	s**t**ay	t	**t**urn
x	**sh**e	zh	**j**unk
ch	**ch**urch or nur**tu**re	sh	**sh**irt
r	leis**ure**	z	rea**ds** or su**ds**
c	ha**ts**	y	fl**ee** or **yea**
a	f**a**ther	o	s**aw**
e	h**er**	i	s**ee**
u	r**u**de	er	**are**
ai	**eye**	ei	**ei**ght or h**ey**
ia	as**ia** or **ya**rd	ie	**ye**s
ang	g**ang**	eng	s**ung**

ABOUT THIS BOOK

INTENDED AUDIENCE

This book will teach you functional practices for the Chinese martial art known as Baguazhang (Eight Trigram Palm). You will learn about the history of the art and the cosmological concept that gives Baguazhang its name.

Martial art practice is more than the study of physical movement. It is an exploration of the mind through the body, and conversely the body through the mind. This book stresses that connection to fulfill practical and spiritual growth.

There are two types of readers that will find this book useful: Those seeking a fitness program that is more than just running and jumping about, and those seeking to improve their martial art practice.

The first type of reader is interested in a fitness program that encourages self development. This reader has tried fitness programs before and abandoned them as boring repetitions of strenuous activity. For this reader, this book presents a complete program that you can apply at your own pace.

When you complete this book, you will have a lifelong program of self development that will not grow stale or become trivial to you. Space and time will not be a factor because you can practice anywhere, anytime, and define your own development.

The second type of reader is familiar with the martial arts and seeks improvement or better understanding of their practice. For this reader the concepts are familiar, but they are unsure of their growth and seek additional material.

Selling martial arts as a method for self defense has been popular in the West--especially in the United States--for the past 40 years. The time and training needed to apply the martial arts in fighting is greater than the average reader is ready to undertake. (A casual scan of the day's headlines reveals that violent crime involves deadly weapons that even the legendary figures of the past could not overcome.)

Readers looking for a *good fight* will find benefit in this book, but only if they are ready to explore beyond the physical aspects of martial art practice.

BOOK DESIGN

As the title implies this book has three components. Each component illustrates an aspect of martial training.

Earth Dragon Canon (Di Long Jing) is a popular phrase in martial art training that commonly refers to ground fighting. *Dragon* (Long) implies fighting forms and *Earth* (Di) meaning on the ground. *Canon* (Jing) means a general principle by which something is judged. So, *Earth Dragon Canon* would be the general principle of ground fighting.

In the internal martial art of Xingyiquan (Form Mind Fist), Earth Dragon Canon is also associated with a circle walking practice called the *twisted root*. Here, *Earth Dragon* implies a circle walking practice that teaches balance, rooting, and fighting skill.

This book borrows from both definitions, but de-emphasizes fighting skill for ground exercises that highlight key internal martial art training methods.

EARTH

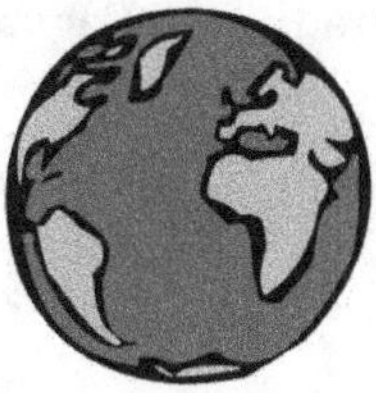

The Earth sections of this book are marked with the above icon. In these sections you will find isometric exercises that you can use to understand key points from the traditional internal martial art teaching, while improving your general fitness. At the end of the book, I combine these exercises into the Internal Power Set formulated around the Taijiquan (Grand Ultimate Fist) classics. This is not a traditional Qigong sequence, but an isometric set that will remind you how the muscles of the body work together to perform the most amazing feat in the natural world--walking upright.

DRAGON

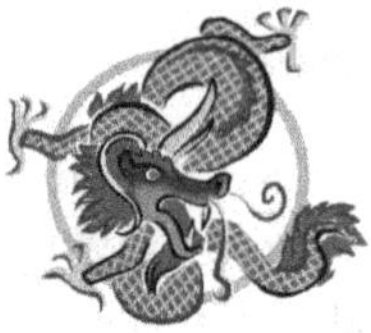

The Dragon sections of the book are marked with the above icon. These sections present the classical training of Baguazhang that includes standing, walking in a circle, and using martial forms when changing directions on the circle.

In the Standing section I introduce four postures that illustrate functional alignment, hand and leg positioning, and key traditional teachings. These postures are referenced repeatedly in the sections that follow; do not ignore them.

After you learn how to stand, the remainder of the book is dedicated to circle walking. These sections include three stepping patterns for walking around the circle, eight Standing Palms, the Single Palm Change, the Double Palm Change, and the Eight Animals from traditional Baguazhang practice.

CANON

The Canon sections of the book are marked with the above icon. *Canon* also means a literary or artistic work considered to be permanently established as being of the highest quality.

Buddhism and Daoism blended into Ch'an--or Zen--Buddhism between the first and sixth centuries CE. Both philosophical systems played an important role in the development of Chinese thought, and the stories of Dong Haichuan--Baguazhang's founder--implies that he developed the art from both lines of thought.

In the Canon sections, I present a historical survey, and a brief summary of both Bagua and Dharma principles that compose the moral character of Baguazhang practice. These sections are introductions for your further study, and I encourage you to look beyond the physical forms and develop a deeper understanding of martial art practice.

LINEAGE TREES

Lineage trees are important to understanding the development of a martial art, but after a few generations they become irrelevant. Lineage trees are used in the breeding of animals where they act as a means of selecting characteristics, and monarchs have used them to prove that their bloodline is pure enough to assume the throne. Unfortunately, many martial art teachers fall into the trap of the latter use, and neglect the importance of the first.

Students who are more concerned with the development of a martial art than the legitimacy of a particular teacher's practice, can follow the lineage tree of certain teachers and see how the martial style developed.

Unfortunately, martial artists that use lineage trees to legitimize their practice are known to exaggerate, or even falsify their lineage. Others become so insistent that a certain lineage is the only one of worth, that they will denigrate the practice methods of other lineages. This makes legitimate research of some martial styles difficult, if not impossible. That is why my efforts center on the work of Sun Lu Tang.

Sun Lu Tang is a constant in martial art study. First, we have his published works. Second, his daughter continued his work and openly shared facts about her father's life, study, and practice. Finally, three separate sources--each with a historical record--identified him as a master of three martial arts.

You can draw similar conclusions about many of Sun Lu Tang's contemporaries. Sun Lu Tang, however, was unique in his efforts to legitimize the boxing arts as self development programs for both the scholar and ruffian.

LEARNING FROM A BOOK

Teaching and learning is like flowing water that can nourish or destroy. Some teachers, or masters, represent martial practice as a path to invulnerability through the magic power of Qi. These teachers are like a raging river that should be avoided and not crossed. Others are only interested in their own learning, or make their practice hard to understand. Others will use flowery terms, with changing definitions, or--worse--claim that the real meaning cannot be known. These teachers are like a wide river that is hard to cross. You may gain understanding, but only with great cost and effort on your part.

There are no secrets in martial art practice. Martial arts are not a path to invulnerability or superhuman powers. Teachers that share the building blocks of proper physical and mental functioning give you the tools for self exploration. These teachers are like a bubbling spring nourishing all who come to drink from it.

Each section in this book has a recommended amount of practice time, but these recommendations are not binding. I want you to develop your own rhythm of practice instead of imposing artificial limits. I also encourage you to read ahead, so you can determine how your practice will develop as you move through the chapters.

The Chinese martial arts intertwine the philosophical concepts of Yin and Yang, Bagua, Wu Xing, and Qi. Understanding the postures' purpose, and the sequence of training includes the study of those concepts. Do not neglect this additional study. Use the Canon sections of this book as a stepping stone to your study.

This is YOUR PRACTICE, take what I give you and make it your own.

There are many books about the practice of martial arts, none--to my knowledge--present the arts as a cohesive mental and physical practice with supplemental exercises. In that respect, I think this book is unique and a first effort on my part. I humbly ask for your feedback on errors and encouragement to continue.

Troy Williams, December, 2008

INTRODUCTION

KNOWING YOURSELF

In the late summer of 1993 I was working for a convenience store chain in Wichita Kansas. During a shift change I kneeled down to open the safe and there was a very loud pop from somewhere below my waist. It was so loud that both the manager I was relieving and the customer he was serving asked, "What was that?"

"I don't know," I replied, "but tell you one thing, I really need to start exercising."

"Exercise. Don't you guys get enough exercise around here," the customer said, "You're going a hundred miles an hour, day and night in this place."

What he said was true enough. The stores I worked for were the busiest in town, and I had worked there for nearly ten years. Those were the days when a single person would run the store for nine or ten hour shifts. During that stretch you would be responsible for taking out the trash, stocking the coolers, making the coffee and tea, and generally keeping the place in shape. When those tasks were complete enough, you would write orders, stock the shelves, and perform general maintenance on anything from a pop machine to a gas pump. It was hard to believe that anyone working at such a job could be out of shape.

I had been thinking about finding an exercise program and *David Carradine's Tai Chi Workout* had earned my attention with a series of infomercials. I had practiced Karate and some Judo in high school, but had never heard of Taijiquan.

The video was about $40 (as I remember) but my wife and I lived on a tight budget, so I would have to take it from cash and be sure we did not miss any bills, making me reluctant to buy the video.

The crack I heard as I opened the safe on that sunny day sealed the deal. That night I bought the *Tai Chi Workout* VHS tape--before the limited offer expired.

The largest part of *David Carradine's Tai Chi Workout* reminded me of middle school calisthenics. Most of the tape was floor exercises followed by something called Qigong. Some of these exercises had exotic names, but were familiar to any gym student. Within a week of starting the program, I was feeling better.

However, learning Taijiquan would have to wait. I had left my longtime employer, and my marriage was failing. We had a high amount of debt on the credit cards, and neither of us was happy. Divorce and bankruptcy were not far off.

When I look back on those darker times, I realize that it was the simple things that brought me through them. BookStar had opened recently, and the store had a wide range of martial art books. The section included books about Taijiquan, Baguazhang, and Qigong. I would sit on the floor in the martial art section and consider if Baguazhang or Qigong were better than Taijiquan. I would page through the books and examine the pictures or line drawings trying to understand this exotic new world.

Because of where and how I grew up, the ideas presented in these books were a new world to me. I grew up in a conservative Mennonite community where eastern philosophies were only discussed in social studies class. My connection to the outside world was the post office. Magazines like Newsweek and U.S. News brought me the world one week at a time. Marvel and D.C. Comics fed my imagination, and the high school librarian ensured that I discovered works by Tolkien, Dostoevsky, and Bradbury. My first vision of Buddhism was a monk setting fire to himself, and my understanding of China formed during the Cold War. (Younger readers may be unfamiliar with the Buddhist connection to the conflict that took place in Vietnam from 1959 to 1975. For more information see: http://tinyurl.com/yfuk95).

At the book store, a man named Dr. Yang, Jwing-Ming had more books on the shelf than other writers. His yellow book--Yang Style Tai Chi--looked as though it must be his own form. However, upon reading a few pages, I discovered that there was another Yang that had created the form and Yang, Jwing-Ming did not claim to be of any relation. Dr. Yang also had a blue book about Qigong and--after sleeping on it--I decided to start with Dr. Yang's blue book.

I bought the yellow book on Taijiquan a few days after my divorce was final. I was heading for bankruptcy, yet I barely noticed the type of trouble I was in. I worked odd hours, and had a physically demanding job, but I would find a set of Qigong to perform from the blue book on workdays, and spent my days off learning Taijiquan from the yellow book.

I would eat and drink and practice Taijiquan under a 40 year old pin-oak tree. My toy poodle would wander around the yard and exchange barks with the squirrels throwing acorns down at her.

I would read--in detail--each posture in the yellow book and then practice the entire sequence from the beginning to that posture. The book's spine was beginning to break, and rain would soak the book even when I tried to shelter it under the pin-oak, so I just broke it apart entirely and put each page in a plastic sheet protector and put the entire thing in a three ring binder.

This manner of practice allowed me to reconnect with myself. For the first time in my life I realized that the physical exhaustion I felt at the end of a day at work was not physical at all; it was emotional, and mental. The time spent under the pin-oak, learning Taijiquan from Dr. Yang's yellow book, was restoring a type of energy to me that I had not known since I was a child.

I wanted to learn more about Taijiquan than even Dr. Yang's yellow book was providing. I could not afford to attend classes at a local martial art school. Instead, I would go to martial art tournaments and watch for things that I could use. At these tournaments, I decided that I am not a fighter and that if practicing in a school meant engaging in that type of activity, then I did not want any part of it. Besides, I was learning from the book and decided that I did not want to hinder my concentration on it with a new set of instructions.

A few years later, the Internet provided a wealth of new material on the internal martial arts. I decided to take a history tour of the internal martial arts by collecting materials on each of the Taijiquan styles. I would spend weeks learning from each new book or video, and then compare that form to ones I had already learned.

I supplemented my practice with translations of the *Dao De Jing* and the *Yi Jing*, and a regular subscription to Marvin Smalheiser's *T'ai Chi Magazine*. The strange world of a few years ago had turned into a vocabulary I used for personal growth.

By mid-2000 I was in a new house with a new bride and looking for new opportunities with my employer. I had always wanted to be a computer programmer and a position to code Java web applications was opening. I had learned the longest sequence in Chinese martial arts from a book and decided that I could do the same with Java.

I spent hours on my laptop reclined in front of the television. I was learning how to code from open source software sites. I returned to work with practices for coding and Java that surprised the veterans on my team and improved our ability to deliver.

Open source software development is a process where you develop a program and share that program--with all its source code--for others to use and improve upon. These programs develop communities, and the communities interact with other open source communities around the world through the Internet. Organizations and software licenses protect the open model.

With such a large community for me to engage in, and with better pay and activities at work coming because of that engagement, I spent less and less time practicing my martial forms. That was when my left hip started to hurt.

RESPONSIBILITY

I had never felt pain like this before. When I was in grade school, I broke my left arm. That was a sudden pain that had gone away, and I knew when it would heal. This new pain was constant, and nothing gave me encouragement that it would pass.

It was painful to sit, and my hip would get stiff and make it difficult to walk when I stood up. I had overstretched myself in the past and thought that I had overdone it in one of my practice sessions. I tried to loosen my left hip and leg with Taijiquan and Xingyiquan sequences that kept me upright and abandoned Qigong or calisthenic exercises entirely.

My hip and leg would hurt for a couple of days, I would work through it, then it would return. I instinctively knew that I needed more movement but was not yet willing to give enough attention to the solution. There were too many things to learn about software development, calling for more hours behind the computer instead of in martial art practice.

Over a couple of months, my hip was getting worse, and I was starting to blame my martial forms. I never considered that sitting all day at my desk and then all night with a laptop was the cause.

By the end of 2002, I was in the type of pain that never quit. I could not sit, lie down, or walk without hurting. I asked friends, family, and coworkers for advice about a doctor and visited a physician. Without some incident to indicate an injury he believed that I was developing arthritis in my hip. I said that it felt like my muscles and not my bones, but he insisted that was common and gave me a popular arthritis drug.

I tried the drug to see whether my pain would subside. Within two days, I was feeling sick. My skin felt itchy everywhere, generally I felt odd, and I had sudden bouts of nausea.

I checked the package details and called the nurse's aid. The conclusion we both made was that I was allergic to the drug and should stop taking it. By now I was missing work because I simply could not sit. Lying on my right side was the only way I could get some relief.

I returned to the doctor who scheduled me for an MRI. I explained that I could not lie on my back long enough for an MRI session. He gave me Lortabs and a quick thinking nurse's aid put my feet up in the air so my back would lie flat on the MRI table.

The pain did not stop. The MRI confirmed that I did not have a slipped disk, and the doctor sent me to a physical therapist. The physical therapist measured my bones, and did some gait analysis. He determined that my left leg was one centimeter shorter than my right. He said that this short leg had caused my hip socket to be stretched further on the left side than on the right, and the constant pulling of the muscles was causing them to seize up in an attempt to pull the joint back into place. The long term remedy, he believed, was to get a special shoe for the left leg to provide balance. In addition, he provided a waist belt that I could pull tightly around my hips to help hold them in place.

I was shocked that such a belt existed. It was a combination of straps and metal hinges that I could use to pull the belt very tightly around my hips. It pinched my skin, but when it was in place I did feel better.

I had to pull the belt so tight that I wore it out within a couple of days. I found a rubber heel lift at a shoe store just a few blocks from my house. I put it inside my shoe, and it provided an extra nine millimeters in height on the left side.

I had ruined my second waist belt, and although I hated wearing such a painful contraption for the rest of my life, I called the physical therapist for another. He said that insurance would not allow him to release another belt, and I would have to start paying for them.

I needed answers that were not coming from the medical profession. No matter how often I measured my left leg, it was always the same length as my right, and holding my hips with levers and straps did not appeal to me. I remembered how only two years ago I was touching the ground in the Snake Creeps Down posture of Yang Style Taijiquan, and now I could barely walk.

What had happened to the physically fit individual that practiced under that pin-oak tree with such determination? I used to impress others with my flexibility, now I was ashamed of my pain. I headed to the bookstore and looked for answers.

My intent was to find a book on anatomy to learn the names and connections of the muscles involved in my pain. With that knowledge I would return to the doctor and argue my case, or I would find an alternative exercise program that promised to restore my hip and reduce my pain. I guessed that some type of Yoga, Pilates, or massage therapy was in order.

I found *Pain Free* by Pete Egoscue, and it just happened to flip open to the hip section. Within a few paragraphs, he described my pain and my situation word for word. After a few more paragraphs there were four simple exercises, postures really, that you do standing up and lying on the floor. These postures let gravity pull your body back into functional alignment and reduce your pain. With your pain reduced, you can begin a normal exercise program and start moving again. The premise of the book--according to the jacket--was that the human body is made for movement, and modern society has starved our body from movement. Sitting, it turns out, is a terrible thing for the human body.

I did not spend any time considering my choices, I snatched the book and headed for the register. My wife--used to me spending hours in the bookstore--had to hurry her choices.

Within a couple of days, I was feeling the type of relief I had not experienced in months. Pain was abating instead of getting worse and I could function again. I performed the Sun Style Taijiquan set, just to see how it felt. I had not practiced anything for over a month, and it was good to be with my old friend again. I promised, this time it would be different; I would not sacrifice my God given right to movement for career or monetary gain.

I had a new weapon in my fight for personal growth. The first three chapters of *Pain Free* reopened my eyes to the genius of those old martial art masters. I had studied a wide range of martial forms and focused new skills and understanding into a few forms that I enjoyed most. I had neglected basic calisthenics for some exotic--and some practical--Qigong sequences. Try as you might to avoid them, push-ups and sit-ups are required exercise. I remembered that my introduction to Taijiquan was *David Carradine's Tai Chi Workout,* and that most of the tape was middle school calisthenics done on the floor. I started to integrate a wide range of isometric exercises into my practice. This became so successful and enlightening that I deserted the esoteric Qigong sequences entirely. I linked the isometric floor practices to postures from the martial forms and found that my personal awareness improved dramatically.

FOUNDATIONS

COSMOLOGY

Cosmology is an account or theory of the origin of the Universe, and by extension man's place in it.

Cosmologies often borrow from one another creating new cosmologies by applying the scientific discoveries of the day. Some cosmologies develop into religious beliefs; others develop through the lens of scientific thought.

Here is a quick historical tour of cosmologies:

Brahmanda from the Hindu Rigveda (1500 - 1200 BCE) said that the Universe is a cosmic egg that cycles between expansion and total collapse. It claimed that the Universe is a living entity bound to the perpetual cycle of birth, death, and rebirth.

The Ptolemaic universe (200 CE) said that the Universe orbits around the Earth. It was the model accepted by many world religions of the time.

During the next 1200 years, the Ptolemaic universe graduated through many models until Copernicus turned the Universe inside out and discarded the Earth centric view.

From the time of the Copernican model in 1543 until Einstein in 1917 new models came with scientific discoveries. These included the Kant/Lambert model of matter being endlessly recycled that sounds suspiciously like the Hindu model. After Einstein's relativity theory the number of cosmological models accelerated with the ability of modern instruments to provide detailed measurements of our environment.

Today, we have many choices dueling it out, including String theory, the Uniformly Expanding theory, Big Bang/Big Crunch theory, and--my new favorite--Null Physics.

Baguazhang takes its name from the Daoist cosmology that is classically attributed to Fu Xi. It is a foundation to eastern thought, and--as I related in the Introduction--was a new world to me when I started studying the internal martial arts.

In this section, I introduce three original cosmologies that contributed to the development of China. More than cosmologies, these systems became a way of thinking, forming governments, and making a living. These systems are Daoism, Confucianism, and Buddhism. Individually, or in concert, they have left an imprint on Asian martial arts.

I introduce these cosmologies as a survey of Chinese history, because such discussions often present the classical Chinese cosmologies as ideas that are fixed in time, or in polar opposition to each other. This view is further enforced through popular culture--such as martial art movies--where conflict between Buddhist, Daoist, and Confucian thought is emphasized as a storytelling mechanism. When viewed through the long lens of history, however, you find that these systems borrowed from each other as they influenced China's development.

This section provides a framework for your further studies. The section starts before the birth of China when Buddha, Confucius, and Laozi were laying down the philosophical systems that would shape the nation. After China organizes as an empire, philosophers, historians, and government officials reflect on this golden age. Some choose Daoism as the example of perfect life, others Buddhism, and others Confucianism. Dynasties rise and fall, and each system has its limelight, only to be replaced by another in a few years.

Because of this constant turmoil, no one system made it to the modern age without taking on characteristics of the others. The first example of this adaptability was Confucius himself, who took the Yi Jing--a Daoist text filled with superstition--and turned it into a manual on proper living. Then, during a period of turmoil, Buddhism--an already adaptable system--absorbed Daoism, and the Zen branch of Buddhism sprang from Bodhidarma and the Shaolin Temple.

ORIGINS

In the beginning there was nothing but a formless chaos. Out of this chaos, there was born an egg. When the egg split the heavy yolk sank to become the Earth, while the light egg white rose to become the Heavens.

The idea that the Universe is made of two forces, a heavy Yin aspect and a lighter Yang aspect whose separation and interaction are constantly creating all aspects of the Universe, is the foundation of Daoism. This line of thought developed to include all the social, and physical interactions of man.

Before it developed into a complex system of creation and organization, Daoism was more practical--Yin and Yang representing different times of the day and of the year. Daylight was the time for work, night was for rest.

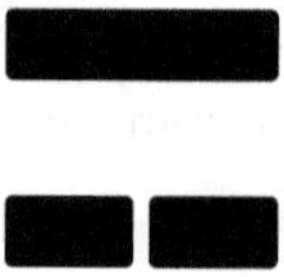

Yin and Yang are represented by two lines. Yang is a solid line that represents brightness, lightness, masculinity, and the tendency to move upwards. Yin is a broken line that represents darkness, heaviness, the feminine, and the tendency to move downwards.

Yin is a time to plant and rest, while Yang is time for harvesting and working. Being in accord with nature meant living into the next year, and if your crops did well then you might prosper from your good virtue.

Fu Xi is a cultural hero reputed to have taught the Chinese people the skills needed to form a civilization. He is depicted

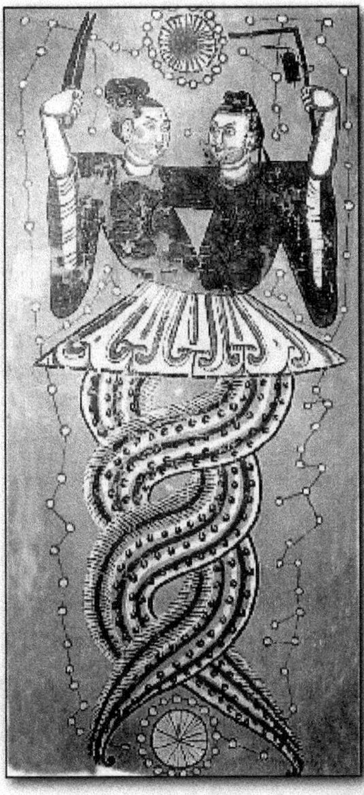

Nuwa and Fu Xi

with his female predecessor the goddess Nuwa. They are holding a compass and a square, further illustrating the complementary, and yet opposite forces of Yin and Yang.

In 2852 BCE Fu Xi is also credited with creating the Eight Trigrams (Bagua), which forms the basis of the *Book of Changes* (*Yi Jing*). The trigrams of the Bagua, and the hexagrams of the *Yi Jing* are more complex representations of the simple Yin and Yang symbols of a broken and solid line. Chinese calligraphy developed from these representations. (*See* Appendix--Trigram Associations for the names and associations of the eight Bagua trigrams.)

He further developed the eight trigrams into an arrangement that was revealed to him on the back of a turtle that emerged from the Yellow River.

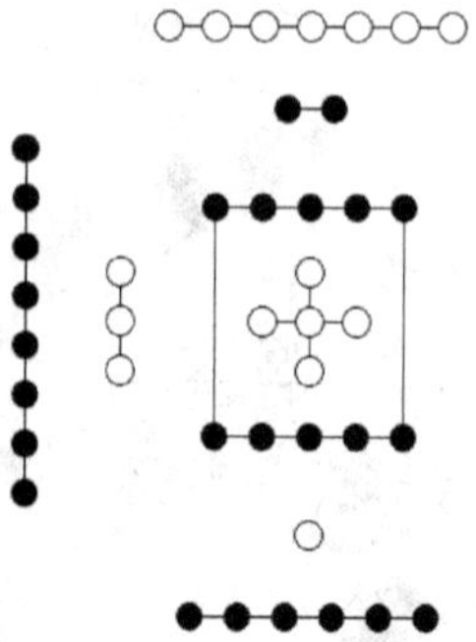

The River Map

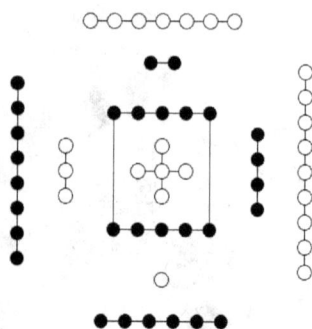

The dots are unitary (base one) representations of the integers one through ten. In this diagram the sum of all the odd or even integers on the periphery equal 20. Adding any number on the inside squares with 5 (the center) will equal the number on the outer square. A modern representation looks like a cross with ten and 5 in the center.

		7			
		2			
8	3	10 5	4	9	
		1			
		6			

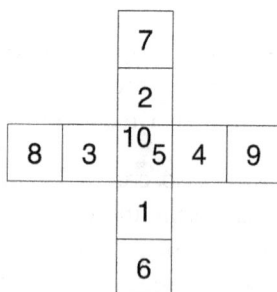

The legend says that Fu Xi created the pre-heaven Bagua circle from his understanding of this arrangement.

In this arrangement the trigrams across from each other represent opposites, much like the even and odd numbers oppose

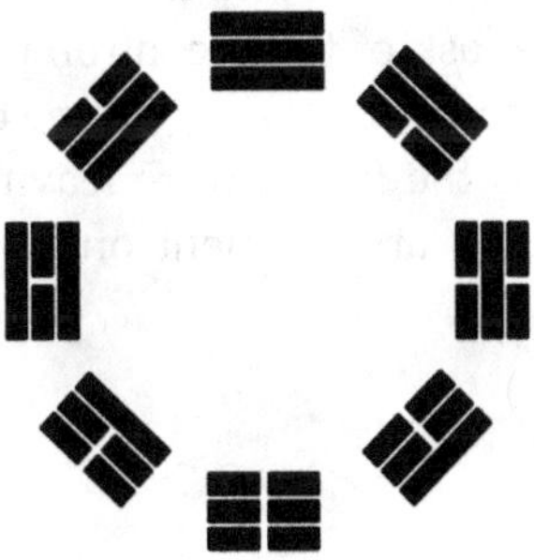

Pre-Heaven Bagua

each other on the diagram. A later method of divination associated the numbers on the outer edge of this arrangement to four possible values, or conditions, of Yin and Yang (6, 7, 8, 9 correspond to Old Yin, Young Yang, Young Yin, and Old Yang).

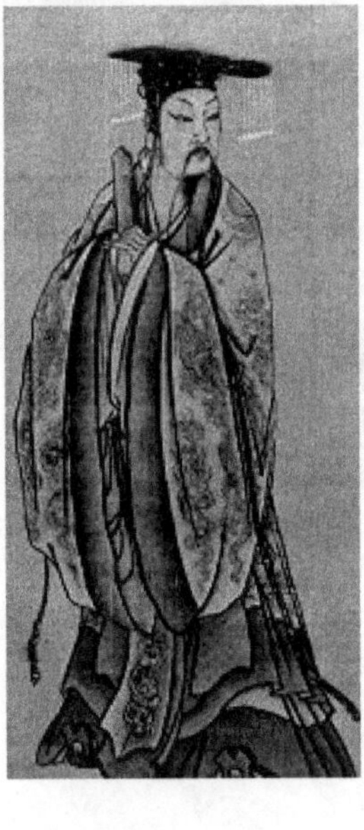

Yu the Great

Another legend associates the arrangement of the trigrams to Yu the Great. Yu is regarded as the founder of the Xia Dynasty (2205 - 1600 BCE) and inventor of flood control techniques. Yu was dedicated to the task of flood control, passing by his house three times without going in, saying that he could not rest in his own home as long as the floods were leaving others homeless. He reportedly saw this arrangement on the back of a tortoise from the Lou River.

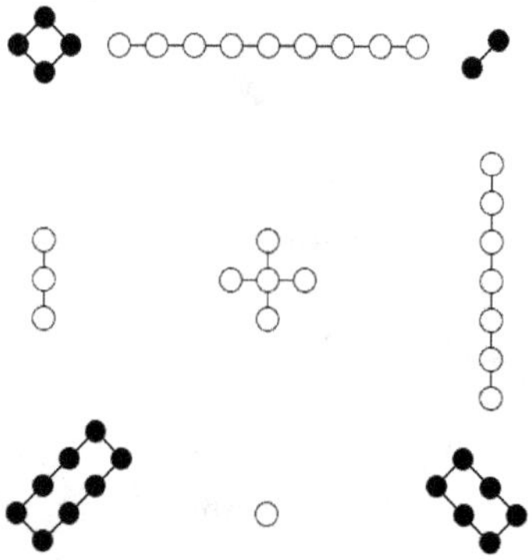

Lou River Scroll

The dots are unitary (base one) representations of the integers one through nine. The odd and even numbers alternate in the periphery of the pattern, the four even numbers are at the four corners, and the five odd numbers form a cross in the center of the square. The sums in each of the three rows, in each of the three columns, and in both diagonals, is 15. Fifteen is the number of days in each of the 24 cycles of the Chinese solar calendar. Since five is in the center, the sum of any two cells that are opposite each other is 10. The pattern's modern representation is a magic square.

4	9	2
3	5	7
8	1	6

QI AND THE FIVE ELEMENTS

Before Yu, however, there was Huangdi--The Yellow Emperor (2497 - 2398 BCE)--the inventor of Chinese medicine. In his classic work the *Huangdi Neijing* (*Yellow Emperor's Inner Canon*) the Universe is composed of various principles, such as Yin and Yang, Qi, and the Five Phases (Wu Xing). The work was one of the first medical treatise to stress the integration of both spiritual and physical treatments as a holistic approach to medical treatment.

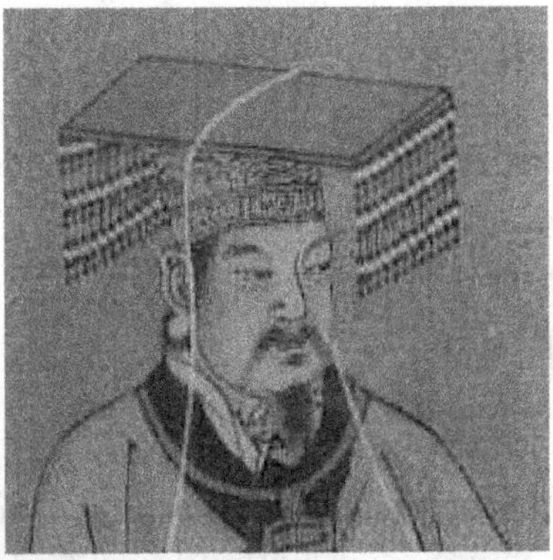

Huangdi - The Yellow Emperor

The *Huangdi Neijing* is composed of two texts. The first text--*Suwen*, or *Basic Questions*--covers the theoretical foundation of Chinese medicine and its diagnostic methods. The *Suwen* includes topics on Feng Shui, Qigong, acupuncture, herbal medicine, fortune telling, meteorology, and astrology. Because of this vast amount of information it is a major text of Daoism. The second text--*Lingshu*, or *Spiritual Pivot*--shares the practical elements of acupuncture therapy in great detail.

The *Huangdi Neijing* is the earliest reference, I could find, detailing the Five Phases, or Five Elements theory. The Five Phases are Wood, Fire, Earth, Metal, and Water. These phases are not elements, but relationships, and interactions between phenomena, especially Qi. These phases create, destroy, and oppose one another. Each phase is affiliated with various aspects in nature and the human body. (*See* Appendix--Five Phases Associations and Appendix--Five Phases Diagram for these relationships and interactions.)

In the *Suwen* Qi is part of everything that exists, as a life force or spiritual energy that pervades the natural world. The Universe does not exist as a series of discrete entities but as a relationship between Yin and Yang and the Five Phases. When Yin and Yang or the Five Phases transform they do so through the emotive force of Qi.

Note that this cosmology addresses the question of change in both the outer world of the cosmos and the inner world of the human body, without regard to a creator. The world is one interconnected whole, where everything and every being moves and acts in a certain way that can either agree or contend with the greater flow, or Dao.

The *Suwen* asserts that Qi circulates through channels in the human body known as meridians. In this context air Qi combines with grain Qi (or food) to produce gathering Qi. When gathering Qi combines again with original Qi (or essence) normal Qi is produced. Normal Qi is divided again into two components--nutritive and defensive. When the body becomes ill, Qi is described as deficient, sinking, stagnant or rebellious. The symptoms of illness are the products of this bad Qi. You can restore balance by adjusting the Qi flow with a variety of therapeutic techniques, including acupuncture, moving to a different location, changing your diet, or the physical practice of Qigong.

POST-HEAVEN BAGUA

When Jou the Terrible ascended to the throne of the Shang dynasty (1600 - 1122 BCE), his behavior was so horrific that his name is synonymous with "a debauched tyrant." Meanwhile, the nearby state of Zhou was gaining influence and the neighboring states would bring their disputes before King Wen of Zhou (1099 - 1050 BCE) to be settled since they knew King Wen provided a wise and fair arbitration.

On one of King Wen's visits to the Shang court, Jou the Terrible threw him in prison, where he was confined for seven years. While in prison, King Wen reflected on Yin and Yang, the Five Phases, and the trigrams of the Bagua. He decided to stack one trigram upon another trigram to form a hexagram--symbolizing a higher level of diversification. He attached a name and a description to each of the sixty-four possible hexagrams. He also rearranged the trigrams on the Bagua circle to reflect the complexity of the natural world--including the change of seasons and the interaction of the Five Phases. This arrangement is the post-heaven Bagua circle.

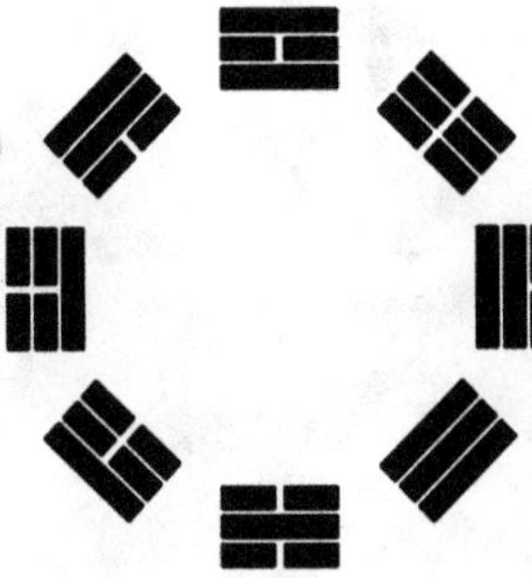

Post-Heaven Bagua

King Wen died before Jou could be overthrown, but his legacy would live on as the Zhou dynasty. The next 800 years would be known as the Golden Age of Philosophers.

UNCARVED BLOCK

If Laozi (Lao Tzu)--the old sage usually associated with Daoism--existed, he lived in this Golden Age. The book attributed to him--*The Way and Its Virtue* (*Dao De Jing*)--represents the ideal man living agreeably with nature.

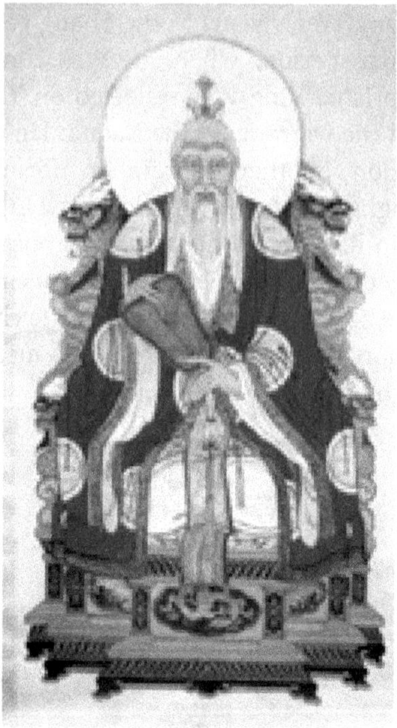

Laozi

Laozi was probably a librarian in the Zhou dynasty Hall of Records. Realizing the dynasty was failing, Laozi headed off to retire in the wild west. At the western border of the kingdom, a guard recognized him as a great philosopher and asked him to share his teachings. The *Dao De Jing* is the result of this conversation.

The *Dao De Jing's* central concepts are Wu Wei, De, and Pu.

Wu Wei is *effortless action* and is associated with water. Water is soft, but through its unrelenting nature can move earth and carve stone. The Way (Dao) of the Universe works on its own rhythm. Individuals striving to form their own way disrupt this rhythm, and pay the price through suffering and an early death.

De is *virtue* or *integrity* and is the active expression of *effortless action.* Aligning your efforts with the unrelenting flow of the Universe is virtuous behavior.

Pu is the *uncarved block,* or *simplicity.* Pu represents a state of receptiveness, without preconceptions, and is the true nature of mind when it is unburdened by knowledge or experiences. Pu is achieved through *effortless action.*

This philosophy of virtue through natural action would have a profound influence on Chinese thought.

HARMONIOUS SOCIETY

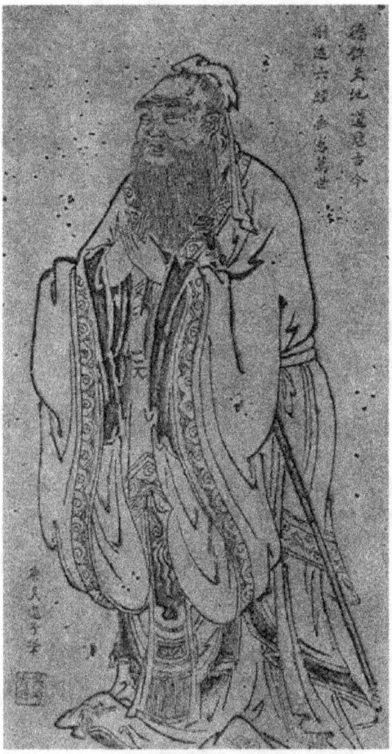

Confucius

Confucius (551 - 479 BCE) taught personal and public morality, correctness of social relationships, justice and sincerity. Confucius hated disorder and disunity and wanted to find ways to overcome the feuds that characterized the latter part of the

Zhou era. He admired King Wen, valued continuity and wanted to sustain the ancient traditions. He tried--unsuccessfully--to persuade many different rulers to put his social and political beliefs into practice. He died convinced that he had failed.

According to Confucius there is a hierarchical external social order, which is mirrored by a personal internal order. Development of both the state and the individual can be likened to the structures of the hexagrams of the *Yi Jing*. He reflected this understanding by attaching commentaries to the hexagrams of the *Yi Jing* known as *The Ten Wings*.

Before Confucius' commentary the *Yi Jing* was used primarily for divination. After his addition the text transformed into a work that has inspired philosophers and scientists for centuries.

In 221 BCE Qin Shi Huangdi assumed *The Mandate of Heaven* and became the first emperor of China. He considered the idle pursuit of philosophy a threat to his throne and has 300 Confucian scholars buried alive. Fortunately, the Qin rule lasts a mere 15 years, when it is replaced by the Han.

The Han was the longest lived imperial dynasty (24 emperors, 426 years). During its rule *The Ten Wings* of the *Yi Jing* and other Confucian texts became templates for state policy.

THE EIGHTFOLD PATH

Buddhism is based on the teachings of Siddhartha Gautama (563 - 483 BCE) who--through a period of exploration--became The Buddha, or Awakened One. He lived in the northeastern region of the Indian subcontinent, but his teachings helped to shape China's development.

Buddhists recognize Gautama Buddha as an awakened teacher who shared his insights with others. These teachings describe the true origins of suffering, and how to overcome them. With this understanding the individual can achieve *nirvana*. Nirvana is a transcendent state in which there is no suffering, and the subject is released from the effects of karma (the sum of a person's actions) and samsara (the cycle of death and rebirth). Nirvana represents the final goal of Buddhism.

Buddhism is broadly categorized into two major branches: The Theravada and the Mahayana schools.

The Theravada school is known as *The Ancient Teaching,* and is considered the oldest surviving Buddhist school. Theravada practice puts importance on monastic life. Religious attainment is an exclusive domain of the bhikkhus (religious renunciants). The arhat (monk) is a person who successfully follows the historical Buddha's teachings. In this practice, it may take many lifetimes before nirvana is attained.

The Mahayana school has a large religious and philosophical structure. Unlike the Theravada school, Mahayana teaches that liberation is universal and not exclusive to religious renunciants. It says that pursuing the release from suffering and attainment of nirvana is too narrow an aspiration because it lacks the motivation to liberate others.

In the Mahayana school emphasis is on becoming a bodhisattva. A bodhisattva is someone that gains *enlightened* (bodhi) *existence* (sattva), but rejects nirvana for teaching others. The bodhisattva has a considerable degree of understanding and uses their wisdom to help others free themselves.

Gautama Buddha abandoned practices of asceticism or self-indulgence that were popular paths to enlightenment for his day. Instead he opted for a *middle way,* or a path of moderation, whose defining characteristic was meditation. His teachings are summarized in The Four Noble Truths and Eightfold Noble Path.

The Four Noble Truths:

1. *The truth of suffering* teaches that life and everything in it is suffering. From birth through death beings are in contact with what they dislike and separated from what they desire.

2. *The truth of the cause of suffering* teaches that suffering is caused by selfish craving. Discomfort and suffering are not the same thing. We suffer in the mind from our attachments to things and ideas.

3. *The truth to the end of suffering* teaches that selfish craving can be overcome with the realization that suffering begins and ends in the mind.

4. *The true path to end suffering* teaches us to live in a harmless way by following the Eightfold Noble Path.

The Eightfold Noble Path:

1. Right Understanding: Understanding the origin of suffering and its extinction as outlined in the Four Noble Truths.

2. Right Thought: Be free of attachment, ill will, views and opinions. Direct the mind towards benevolence and kindness.

3. Right Speech: Abstain from lying, gossiping, and speaking unnecessarily or harshly.

4. Right Action: Abstain from killing, stealing, and immorality.

5. Right Livelihood: Maintain one's livelihood without harming living beings.

6. Right Effort: Remain aware and unattached in all circumstances.

7. Right Mindfulness: Be aware of all that one does in speech, action, and thought.

8. Right Concentration: Be free of mental disturbances such as worry, anxiety, or envy. To be at one with life in this moment.

Buddhism did not appear suddenly in China; rather it grew gradually during periods of turmoil. At first, Buddha was seen as a barbarian god, favored by the non-Chinese ruling in the North. Buddhism saw growth during hard times as the self-denying life of Buddhist monks appealed to peasants subjected to increasingly despotic rule. The monks would live and work among the people, instead of cloistered away like the elite Confucian scholars.

Buddhist monks, imported from India, embraced the ideals of Confucianism and Daoism so successfully that a new branch of the belief system--Ch'an or Zen--was born.

ZEN

Bodhidharma (440 - 534 CE), a bodhisattva who traveled to China during the Period of Disunion (220 - 581 CE), played a seminal role in the transmission of Mahayana Buddhism from India to China.

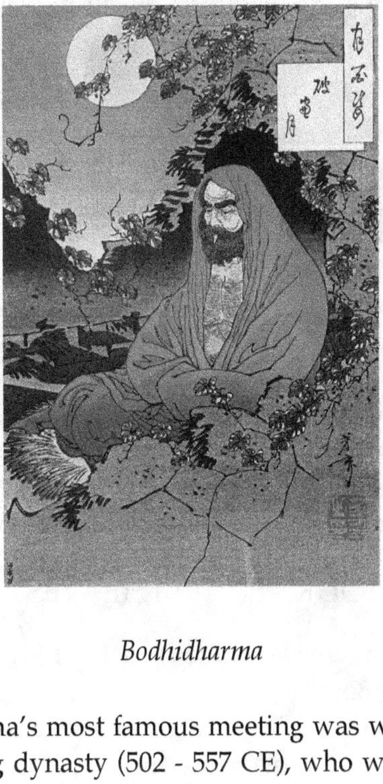

Bodhidharma

Bodhidharma's most famous meeting was with the emperor Wu of the Liang dynasty (502 - 557 CE), who was a strong supporter of Buddhism. The emperor Wu asked Bodhidharma how much merit his building of temples, printing of scriptures, and support for the Buddhist community had accumulated. Bodhidharma replied, "No merit at all." The Emperor then asked Bodhidharma, "What is the highest meaning of the holy truths?" Bodhidarma replied, "Without holiness." The emperor Wu then demanded to know who Bodhidharma was to say such things. Bodhidharma responded, "I don't know." Incensed by Bodhidharma's answers the emperor Wu had him expelled from the court.

Bodhidharma traveled north, across the Yangtze River. He stopped at the Shaolin temple at Mt. Song but was refused entry. Legend says that he sat in meditation outside the monastery, facing its walls, for nine years. The monks were impressed with his dedication and granted him entry to the monastery. Once inside, he was dismayed by the poor physical condition of the monks and began teaching a set of exercises to the monks to promote their physical health.

This legend says that those exercises were the 18 Arhat Hands of Shaolin--a common routine in Shaolin martial arts. It is more likely that these exercises were yoga postures that were mixed with an already developed martial tradition to form the Shaolin arts.

Bodhidharma's transformative presence at the Shaolin temple was a keystone moment that forever changed martial training. Mankind had always trained to fight--initially to defend himself from animals or to hunt large game--and the Chinese were using form routines in martial practice before Bodhidharma. What changed at the Shaolin temple, is the use of martial training as a form of physical exercise.

JOURNEY TO THE WEST

In 581 the emperor Wendi (541 - 604 CE) reunified China as the Sui dynasty. Born as Yang Jian in a Buddhist temple Wendi gained the support of elite Confucian scholars and made Buddhism a central pillar of his new dynasty.

The Tang Dynasty (618 - 649 CE), however, would deliver an early threat to Buddhism in China. The emperor Taizong (626 - 649 CE) said that the Buddha "was a crafty barbarian who deluded his own countrymen," and "It is not that I do not understand Buddhism, but rather that I despise it, and refuse to study it." When Xuan Zhang--a Chinese Buddhist monk--returned from his perilous trip to India with 657 sutras on his back and an epic story to tell, Taizong had a change of heart, and took the monk as his spiritual teacher. Xuan Zhang also left a book, Records of the Western Regions, which became the basis for the classic saga, Journey to the West.

Written during the later Ming dynasty, *Journey to the West* referred to the journey of Xuan Zhang in a fictional manner. The novel includes three fantastic disciples of the Buddhist monk, Sun Wukong (Monkey King), Zhu Baijie (Eight Precept Pig), and Sha Wujing (Friar Sand). Their mythical trip to India is an allegory for enlightenment. The story is steeped in Buddhist and Daoist morality and is a satire of Ming Chinese bureaucracy.

ZHANG SANFENG

Zhang Sanfeng (1247 - 1370) is another legendary figure of Daoism, and the mythical creator of Taijiquan. Some stories about Zhang Sanfeng place him as early as the Five Dynasties and Ten Kingdoms period (907 - 960 CE) when China was undergoing another period of disunion. Others place him in the Song dynasty (960 - 1279 CE) which saw many achievements in science, philosophy, and arts, including the first use of printing (700 years before it was used in Europe), and the use of gunpowder (invented by Daoists during the Tang dynasty) in grenades.

If Zhang Sanfeng existed he was probably born in 1247 and lived during the years of Marco Polo's (1254 - 1324 CE) visit to China. He studied Buddhism and martial arts at the Shaolin temple before leaving and establishing the Daoist temples at

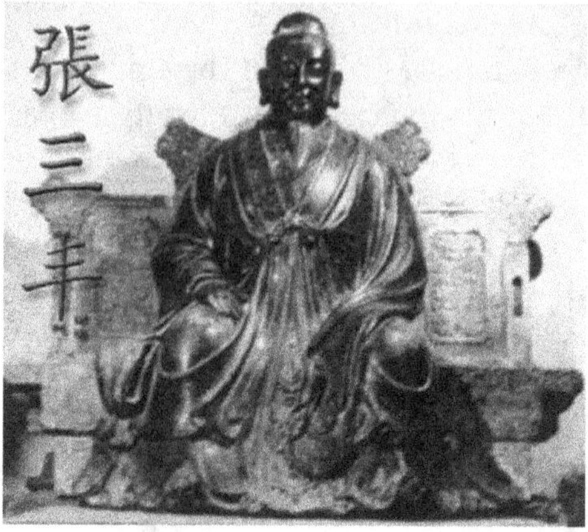

Zhang Sanfeng

Wudang Mountain. It was at Wudang Mountain that Zhang Sanfeng created the martial art of Taijiquan. The story says that he saw a magpie and serpent fighting in the grass. He considered the softness and fierceness of both creatures, and incorporated these ideas with his knowledge of the *Huangdi Neijing,* and Shaolin martial arts to form Taijiquan.

YUE FEI

Yue Fei (1103 - 1142 CE) was a great military leader who is credited with the creation of many Qigong and martial forms including Xingyiquan, Eight Pieces of Brocade, and Eagle Claw Boxing. As a child he learned Shaolin martial art from a man who had studied at the Shaolin temple. He also studied the *Art*

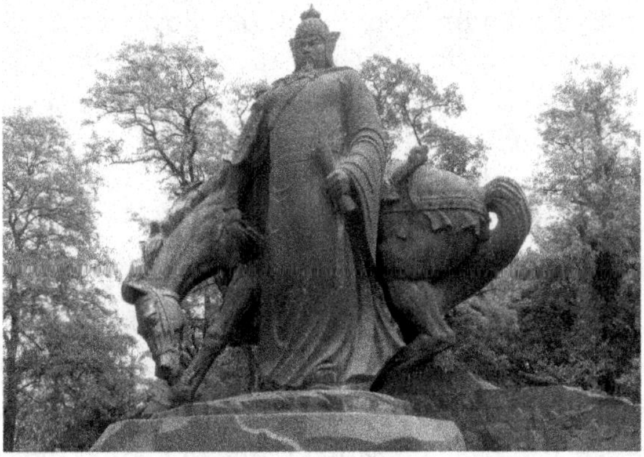

Yue Fei

of War, and other Daoist texts. During this period, Jurchen invaders threatened to overthrow the Song dynasty. Since Yue Fei carefully chose, conditioned, and trained his army--with the aforementioned forms--he was very successful on the battlefield. He was ready to launch a major assault on the Jurchen invaders when court officials conspired to have Yue Fei killed. The story of his betrayal became legend during the Ming dynasty when a book which refers to this story, *Tale of the Eastern Window,* became popular.

FALL OF EMPIRE

In 1644 the Manchus marched into Beijing and formed China's last dynasty, the Qing (1644 - 1912). The Manchus were an ethnic minority, and forced the Han majority to shave the fronts of their heads and wear pigtails as a sign of submission.

The Qing period was marked with political intrigue as China's borders were put under increasing pressure by Western powers. A failure to modernize politically and economically ended the Chinese empire after more than two millennia. In a strange twist, that fall was linked to China's rich martial art tradition.

After a series of natural disasters, and the people being upset by Anglo-French occupation, the Boxer Movement (1890 - 1900 CE) started in rural China. These *spirit boxers* claimed to have built up their Qi with physical exercises and magic charms that gave them invulnerability to bullets. The boxers stormed churches and killed foreigners as the movement gathered strength and moved on Beijing in 1900.

Cixi--the mother of the emperor and dowager empress of China--took control of the country when the emperor died of smallpox. She sided with the Boxer Movement, declaring war on the occupying forces. When the boxers failed to oust the occupying forces she fled Beijing, fearing for her life. After the failure of the Boxer Movement Russia, Germany, France, and Britain divided the country amongst themselves with treaties that did not fully dissolve until the end of the twentieth century.

Sun Yat-sen, a revolutionary leader, took control of China on January 1, 1912. For the next 40 years China would try to copy the government of the United States before the communist revolution in 1949.

ORIGINS OF BAGUAZHANG

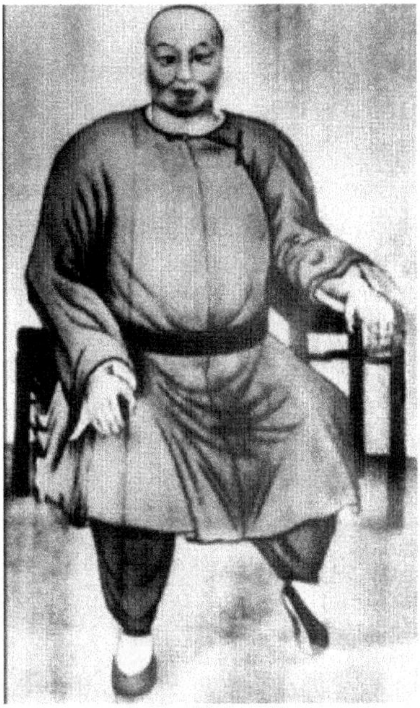

Dong Haichuan

The creation of Baguazhang as a formalized martial art is attributed to Dong Haichuan (1797 - 1882). When discussing the creation of a formalized martial art, identifying the actual events that contributed to its development is difficult. Fanciful stories cast the art as the creation of a legendary figure, or as the secret teachings of a reclusive master. In the case of Dong Haichuan, he was a bit of each--legendary and historical.

The widely accepted historical account of Baguazhang's development says that Dong was a member of the Quanzhen (Complete Truth) sect of Daoism. The Complete Truth Daoist walked in a circle while chanting as a method of meditation.

Dong Haichuan loved to practice martial arts, and he was skilled in Bafanquan (Eight Rotating Boxing). He synthesized

Bafanquan's straight line techniques with circle walking to form his own art called Turning Palm.

Around 1864, Dong arrived in Beijing and gained employment at the Su Wang Palace. After an impressive demonstration of his agility the noble asked him to train household servants in his martial art. Later, Prince Su sent him and his disciple--Yin Fu--to collect taxes in Mongolia. When he returned, he left the Prince's household, and began to teach publicly.

During this later period Dong Haichuan renamed his art to Baguazhang, and the legend of Dong and his creation begins.

In the legendary story, Dong Haichuan was either a criminal or rejected by his father because of a misunderstanding. Forced out of his hometown because of this disgrace, he was wandering the mountains of Hebei province when he came across a Daoist and Buddhist monk practicing circle walking. In some versions, the monks are so skilled in their practice that they can walk on water. Because of his love of martial arts Dong Haichuan wishes to learn the skill of these monks. He manages to gain discipleship with them and trains with them for many years. He leaves the mountains and arrives in Beijing where he gains employment at the Su Wang Palace.

One night, Dong Haichuan was serving drinks at a palace party. The palace was crowded with people, and he couldn't get through the throng to get more drinks. Dong used the *lightness* skill he had learned from the old monks and walked along the walls to get around the crowd. Impressed with Dong Haichuan's skill the noble asked what martial art he practiced. Dong did not have a name for his art so he said that it was Eight Trigram Turning Palm (Baguazhang).

In either case, tales of Dong Haichuan's skill quickly spread and, because of his position at the Su Wang Palace, many experienced martial artists sought him out for instruction. Famous disciples of Dong included Yin Fu--a master of Luohanquan-- and Cheng Tinghua--a master of Shuaijiao. Instead of asking these masters to forget their earlier arts, Dong encouraged them to integrate their previous practice with the circle walking skill.

Because Baguazhang is founded on the *Yi Jing's* core principle of change, there is endless variety to Baguazhang practice. Some schools create routines, others teach only a few postures and encourage spontaneity. All schools, however, teach the basic principle of walking on the circle as the best method for physical health, martial practice, and meditation.

YIN FU

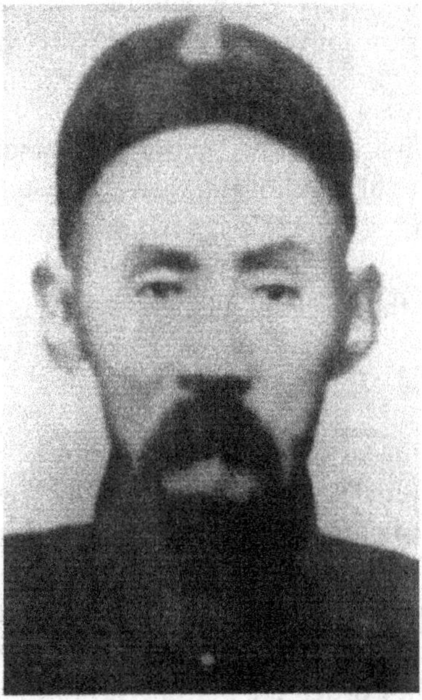

Yin Fu

Yin Fu (1840-1909) was Dong Haichuan's earliest disciple at Su Wang Palace. Some stories say that when he started studying with Dong that he did not appreciate circle walking and focused on striking and kicking methods, even laughing at the circle walking practice. Dong Haichuan was upset at this and said, "If you laugh at circle walking again, you won't have your front teeth any more." Yin Fu began to laugh and Dong used a palm strike to knock out two of Yin Fu's front teeth. After that incident Yin Fu concentrated his practice on the turning palms.

Yin Fu was thin and small, but his strikes were strong, and his circle walking practice made him very fast and agile in a fight. After the incident with Dong Haichuan he studied hard and developed new aspects of the Baguazhang art.

After training with Dong Haichuan, he held a bodyguard office in the imperial palace. Some stories say that he was a personal bodyguard to the dowager empress Cixi, and escorted her from Beijing after the failure of the Boxer Movement.

While acting as a palace bodyguard, Yin Fu also taught martial arts. Yin Fu first taught his students Lohanquan, or Paochui, and only later taught them Baguazhang. Yin Style Baguazhang is known for its strikes, kicks, and unique palm formation known as the ox's tongue. The four fingers are close together, and the thumb pulls into the center of the hand which is hollow.

CHENG TINGHUA

Cheng Tinghua (1848 – 1900) was the fourth disciple of Dong Haichuan. He owned an eyeglass shop in Beijing, so some called him Eyeglasses Cheng. During the Boxer Movement (July 1900) Cheng saw the invading armies killing and looting throughout Beijing. Upset at what was happening to his country, he swore to defend it. One day, Cheng Tinghua subdued ten of the looting soldiers before they ordered a patrol with rifles to surround him.

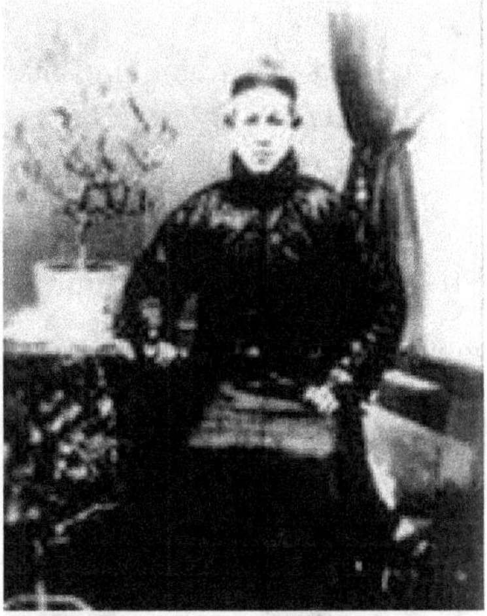

Cheng Tinghua

Cheng used his Baguazhang skills to calmly evade the soldiers and leaped onto a wall where he started to walk away. The soldiers shot him dead.

Before he started studying with Dong Haichuan, Cheng Tinghua had an extensive background in Shuaijiao (Chinese Wrestling); therefore, Cheng Style Baguazhang is known for its throwing techniques. The hand is held in the Dragon Claw formation with the thumb spread wide, the tiger's mouth curved up, the second, third, and fourth fingers are slightly spread apart, and the little finger and fourth finger held together.

SUN LU TANG

Sun Lu Tang (1861-1932) was a renowned master of Chinese martial arts and the creator of Sun Style Taijiquan. He was an accomplished Confucian and Daoist scholar, and contributed to the development of the internal martial arts through his published works.

Sun Lu Tang's first book--*A Study of Form Mind Boxing* (1915)--illustrated the complete training method for Xingyiquan.

In this book he made the argument that literary and martial art learning was the same, and that training in martial arts benefits the health of the practitioner.

His second book--*A Study of Eight Trigrams Boxing* (1916)--was the first book on Baguazhang. In this book, he connected the physical forms to the diagrams and philosophy of the *Yi Jing*.

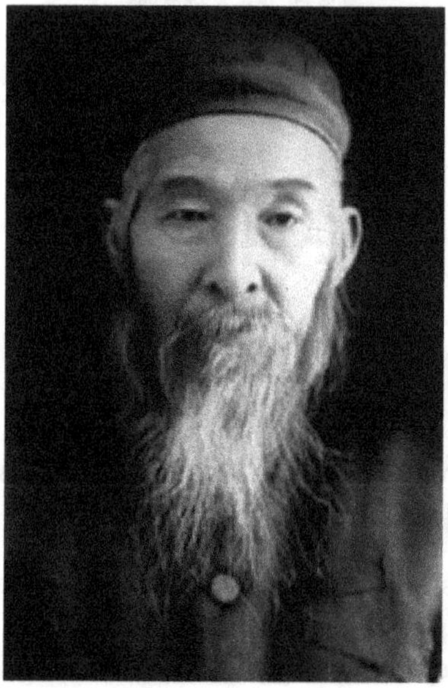

Sun Lu Tang

His third book--*A Study of Grand Ultimate Boxing* (1921)--detailed his own Taijiquan form, and forever categorized the martial arts of Baguazhang, Xingyiquan, and Taijiquan as *internal* martial arts.

It is difficult to determine if the division of Chinese martial arts between *external* and *internal* forms existed before Sun Lu Tang. In his book on Taijiquan he traces the development of martial arts to "ancient times," saying that martial arts were developed to prevent the body from "growing weaker by the day, and the hundred illnesses invading." He further says that exercises created by Bodhidarma at the Shaolin temple were the basis for Yue Fei's and Zhang Sanfeng's martial and Qigong systems.

He joined Yang Chengfu and Wu Chienchuan--of Taijiquan fame--on the faculty of the *Beijing Physical Education Research Institute* where they taught the internal martial arts to the public. He published two more books before his death in 1932.

MARTIAL ARTS

MARTIAL ARTS IN ANGER

In open source software development, there is a phrase "in anger." (Refer to the Introduction for more information about open source software and my experience with it.) "In anger" means that a program or a process was developed out of frustration with what was available. I write this section out of a similar frustration.

The trend in martial art publications is to stress the combat effectiveness of a given art. Even stressing the art's "brutal" nature, claiming that it was born in "combat and violence." For certain, martial arts are "combat training," but unless you are preparing for war, there is no need for that training to be brutal, or even violent. This is not the twelfth or even the nineteenth century when personal disputes were decided with duels to the death.

So it is "in anger" that I approach the definition of martial arts and the reasons to practice them.

THE MARTIAL ARTS PARABLE

Teneke was smaller and slower than all his classmates. On his way to school each morning the bigger kids would take his lunch, and after school they would push him into the dirt as they ran by him. To protect himself, Teneke would avoid playing with the other kids, and hide in his room, reading and watching television.

At night, Teneke would watch the World Fighting Show and dream of having the skills of Bone Cutter--the World Fighting Show champion--so he could beat the bullies, take their lunch, and push them into the dirt. But, the next morning he would walk to school in fear of the bullies, and try to avoid them.

Teneke's great uncle owned a martial art school where he taught the same martial art Bone Cutter bragged about on television.

Sometimes Teneke would sit in on his great uncle's classes and watch the students practice. When he would ask his great uncle to teach him how to fight like Bone Cutter, his uncle would say that is just television and pretend. That no one can fight like Bone Cutter, and that he just does and says those things to make money.

Teneke would insist, and his uncle would finally relent. Instead of teaching Teneke the Splitting Chop that Bone Cutter would use to send his opponents out of the ring, his great uncle would just ask him to stand with his arms up and his legs deeply bent.

Teneke, feeling that he was finally learning his great uncle's martial art would stand for a few minutes, but his legs, and arms would begin to hurt and he would stop. When he would ask to learn something else, his great uncle would just have him go and stand again, saying that he was not ready to learn something new.

Finally, Teneke would just stop and leave the class, thinking that his uncle did not want to teach him.

One day, Teneke tried to resist one of the bullies. He had been watching carefully in his great uncle's class as the students learned the Splitting Chop movement. After a couple of hours of practice, Teneke was sure that he could execute a Splitting Chop to the bully and defeat him.

Instead, the bully punched Teneke in the face, and made his nose bleed. Teneke, feeling humiliated, ran to the martial art school and knocked on the door. His great uncle opened the door and asked what had happened. Teneke explained that a bully had punched him in the nose and made him bleed.

Teneke was crying and blaming his great uncle for not being as skilled as Bone Cutter with his Splitting Chop movement.

"What do you mean?" asked his great uncle.

Teneke explained that he had watched in class and practiced the Splitting Chop movement in secret. But, the bully beat him up anyway.

"Have you been practicing the standing postures I showed you?" his great uncle asked.

Teneke replied that he had not. They were boring, and made his arms and legs hurt. "Can't you just teach me the Splitting Chop movement the way Bone Cutter does it?"

Finally, his great uncle relented and said that, "If you want to learn the Splitting Chop movement, then you must become my disciple."

Teneke was overjoyed, but his great uncle continued, "To be my disciple, you must do all the exercises that I tell you, for as long as I tell you to do them. Do you understand?"

Teneke was so happy to hear that his great uncle would accept him as a disciple, that he agreed to the conditions without realizing that he was just going to be standing around again.

Teneke studied every night after that incident. When his arms and legs would start to hurt, he would remind himself that he was his great uncle's disciple and had to persevere.

As the weeks and months passed, Teneke's health began to improve. He was not the smallest and slowest in his class anymore, and since he was proud to be his great uncle's disciple, he did not try to hide from his classmates. As his health improved, the bullies stopped pushing Teneke down and taking his lunch. Some days, they would even walk with Teneke and he would play games with them after school.

Teneke did not notice this change in the bullies, or his own behavior. He was concerned with his martial art practice and not with taking revenge on the bullies.

Then, one evening, his great uncle asked if Teneke would like to learn the Splitting Chop fist. Suddenly, Teneke remembered why he had been training so hard. Full of understanding, Teneke turned to his great uncle and said, "I don't need to know the Splitting Chop fist, Great Uncle. But, if you show it to me, I will practice it."

With a tear in his eye, Teneke's great uncle began the instruction.

DEFINING MARTIAL ARTS

The New Oxford American Dictionary defines martial art as "various sports or skills, mainly of Asian origin that originated as forms of self-defense or attack, such as judo, karate, and kendo." As the Asian martial arts have grown in popularity, other cultures have shared their own traditions. Notice that while *martial* means *warlike* the definition of the noun *martial art* is a *sport or skill*, not a means of training for war.

I struggled with this definition because it lacked the deeper meaning I have developed in my own marital art practice. After several days of research, meditation, and practice, I realized that what I really wanted to accomplish with this section was not a definition of martial arts, but to define why someone studies martial arts.

Why do I study martial arts? Initially, it was for exercise. As my enjoyment of martial art practice increased, I learned that I needed to look outside the physical practice to find the real reason for my enjoyment. This journey naturally led to the philosophical foundations of Buddhism, Confucianism, and Daoism.

Through this study, I learned that many martial art masters of the past followed a similar journey. They may have come to martial art practice for different reasons, but they all found deeper meaning in their practice. Even when they had mastered the physical practices, they had not mastered the art. They continued their development with the study of Buddhism or Daoism.

In the beginning, all of these journeys are unique. In the end, all of these journeys are the same; the martial art becomes the teacher. A true *martial art* becomes the student's course on self development.

When I say that I am a student of the martial arts, I am not saying that I learned Baguazhang or Taijiquan from this instructor or that grand master. I am saying that the art itself is the instructor. Real study of the martial arts will produce real change in the student beyond improved physical fitness.

COMBAT TRAINING

Many individuals are eager to learn the combat applications of a martial art. Usually, this fascination with combat comes from popular culture, and no real threat. Because martial arts are often marketed as a means of self defense, I feel it is important to explore this subject more closely.

The first question I have for the student seeking to learn the martial arts for combat or self defense is, "Why do you want to know this skill? Are you going to hurt someone?"

Unless you are a psychopath, the answer is no; you do not want to hurt someone, but you may feel unsafe. A feeling to which I have a few more questions: "Why are you afraid? Is it where you live? Is it how you live? Can you change either of those situations before you depend on combat?"

If you can provide heartfelt answers to those questions, and still seek to learn the martial arts for combat, then I ask that you practice five times harder than anyone else. That is, if the practice requires you to stand in a posture for 5 minutes, then you should stand for 25 minutes. If asked to do 25 push ups or crunches, you should do 125. If asked to practice forms (such as walking the circle in Baguazhang) for one hour, then the student seeking real martial skill, honestly seeking to use a martial art for combat, should walk five hours.

Why do I challenge you to such an extreme regimen? Because it takes that type of practice to develop fair skill as a *boxer*. The idea that you can practice an hour a day, with a few minutes of hands-on instruction at the local gym, then defend yourself against an armed and determined criminal, is dangerous. Cheng Tinghua was one of the greatest martial artists ever, and he was shot dead. You will do better?

There is violence and danger in the modern world, but the human race has developed institutions and technologies to enhance individual safety. Take advantage of tools like security alarms, pepper spray and a taser for self defense. Practice martial arts for self development.

Few individuals persist in the type of regimen I outlined above. Most people grow to understand that their images of heroism and violence through martial art training were just that, imagination. With that understanding they are able to take the *middle way* and the art becomes their teacher.

TYPES OF MARTIAL ARTS

The Martial arts of China are divided into two broad categories; external *(waijia)* and internal *(neijia)*. The definition of these two schools varies with distinctions along philosophical and national lines, as well as the type of practice.

The national and philosophical difference started during the Qing dynasty. Remember that the Qing were ethnic Manchus that repressed the ethnic Han majority, even forcing the Han to shave their heads and wear a topknot to distinguish them from the ruling Manchu class. The Shaolin martial arts were defined as external, and associated with the Manchu and Buddhism (imported into China) while internal martial arts were associated with Daoism (indigenous to China). Remember that in the long history of China Daoism and Buddhism were each favored by different emperors. When the Buddhist influence came from forces outside China, it was seen as an inferior system.

Another way to classify an external or internal art is to contrast their methods of practice. External styles train muscular power, speed, and direct martial applications. Most Chinese martial arts are classified as external styles. Internal styles train body connection with awareness of spirit, mind, and breath. Internal martial art training includes standing, stretching, and exercises to improve muscular strength.

In his book on Taijiquan, Sun Lu Tang says that Zhang Sanfeng realized that his Shaolin training caused overexertion from the use of too much strength. This overexertion was causing him physical harm, so Zhang Sanfeng corrected his practice by applying the principles from Bodhidarma's original exercises with the Dao. With this practice, he obtained a smooth and balanced Qi. While few mention the *Huangdi Neijing's* imprint on internal martial art training, preferring to give the credit to Bodhidarma, its influence is evident.

This later definition of an internal martial art allows any martial art, or even any physical training, to become an *internal* practice. By shifting the focus of training from physical (preoccupied with the body and its needs) to physiological (the functions and activities of life) the practice method and purpose changes.

WHY DO YOU PRACTICE?

Baguazhang is classified as an internal martial art. With the understanding you now have about martial arts and the cosmological principles that helped to shape them, you need to decide why you are going to practice Baguazhang. This decision will define *martial art* for you. Once made, this decision is not fixed; it will morph to include different (or even all) aspects outlined below. For now, choose one of these five reasons before continuing:

- *Medical:* You desire to be in better shape, but are not engaged with modern exercise programs. Your practice is based on your current physical condition (no overexertion allowed) with the goal of improving health.

- *Mental:* You feel out of shape mentally. You may feel depressed, cranky, or just have a perplexing problem that you cannot solve. Your practice is focused on breathing and attention with the intent of improving your mood.

- *Spiritual:* You feel that it is time to develop a deeper understanding of yourself and the world around you. In Daoist practice the student seeks to be in harmony with the Dao. The Buddhist practice seeks understanding and enlightenment. A *middle way (Zen),* is to seek enlightenment by following the Dao. (You can associate your practice with any spiritual belief system. You do not have to become a Daoist or Buddhist to practice the martial arts.)

- *Community:* You recognize that engaging yourself and others in physical exercise is one way to improve your community. This idea is not unusual; many Japanese firms, for example, implement a calisthenic routine for their employees. Many studies show that healthy individuals reduce healthcare costs, take fewer sick days, and are more productive.

- *Martial:* The last reason to practice would be the martial one. The purpose of practice is to gain physical power, speed, and skill to overcome an opponent in a fight. The *martial* student is fully engaged in the other four aspects as well, recognizing that real warriors contribute to their community, through physical, spiritual, and mental well being.

ATTENTION

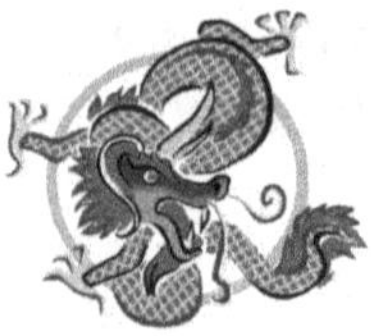

Before you start physical exercise, take a moment to consider if you can engage in the motion requirements of that activity.

You never consider your physical condition when you bend down to pick up a dropped piece of paper, or grab a suitcase from the baggage carousel at the airport. During these innocent movements you will hear the back crack or the hip pop, and you find yourself in the doctor's office seeking relief.

It was not the innocent movement at the office or airport that caused the pain or injury. It was the lack of motion, or the repetition of thousands of other motions that created the conditions for the innocent movement to become a life changing experience. Picking up your luggage, or bending to tie your shoe is a motion that your body can perform. It is a wonderfully designed machine with levers and pulleys all cooperating to perform the most wonderful feat in the natural world--walking upright.

The problem with the modern world is that you do not do enough of this--walking upright--and the cooperation between large and small muscles breaks down. Therefore, before starting this or any exercise program you must perform a careful self examination and ask yourself: "What types of physical activity can I safely do?" Consider the flexibility of your joints and back. If there is pain or tightness in these areas, you may want to consider other exercise programs to repair those conditions before you embark on this journey.

The most important concept you will explore in this book is *attention*. When you say the word attention individuals have different reactions. In the military, it means to stop your current activity and stand at attention. In school, it means to set aside the cell phone or MP3 player and give your full focus to the instructor. In relationships, it means to take notice of someone. We pay attention to problems so that we may correct them. Doctors and

CEOs are blamed for their inattention when a patient dies, or a company fails.

You have paid attention to television, to work, to email, to books, to traffic, to problems and circumstances, to money and occupation, to family, and friends, but have you paid attention to yourself?

Your first exercise is to sit somewhere uncomfortable with no distractions. You need somewhere uncomfortable to break through the mind clutter and help you to become aware of your surroundings. If you start by sitting somewhere comfortable, you will not be able to turn off your random thoughts.

A stairway in or near your home is ideal. Stairs are often narrow and hard enough that if you sit up straight you will be uncomfortable. Choose a position high enough that you can put your thighs out flat in front of you.

You need to turn off the television or radio in the background so you can be quiet and alone for a few minutes. Turn off your cellphone.

You should have absolutely nothing to do while you are sitting. Before you sit down make a note of the time and try not to have any timekeeping device within eyeshot.

Now, sit straight up, trying to eliminate any arch in your back. Place your hands on your thighs and relax your shoulders; try to pull them back a little if you can. Breathe in and out through your nose. Make the breaths long and smooth. You should be intensely aware of your breathing, and nothing else.

Sit. Breathe. Be attentive to yourself. At some point, you will aimlessly get up and continue with the same mindless activities you were doing before you began the exercise. When you notice that is what you have done, take note of the time and determine how long you could be attentive to yourself.

You are not trying to sit for a certain amount of time, but rather long enough to pay back some of that attention you have been paying out to everything else.

Continue this practice for two weeks or a month. Noting how long you can sit each day. It may help your practice to keep a journal. In your journal, you can make a note of how long you can sit each day and what types of activities were happening around you. Note how those things affected your ability to be attentive.

Attention has a high regard in internal martial art practice because it is the key to winning a fight. The slow, careful movements of prearranged practice are less about the form and more about your attention to the moment.

In this case, the fight is adding motion to your life, and the enemies are your unhealthy reactions to obligations, work, and various types of entertainment media. The first step--asking each of those enemies to step aside a few minutes so you can pay some attention to yourself--is crucial. Without creating this initial battle line, your practice will fail and you will find this book on a heap of junk in your next garage sale.

The practice of attention gives the internal martial art student an advantage over other exercise programs. With attention you are less likely to hurt yourself, or someone else. With attention, you understand where you are weak and where you are strong. With attention you can develop your own program of practice that will change with the seasons, your personal experiences, and skill level.

For the internal martial art student, attention means stopping if there is pain (overexertion). The exercises described in this book are as simple as standing and walking. They are not presented as a cure for existing conditions, and they assume a certain level of physical well-being before you begin. If either standing or walking is causing you pain today, then you need help beyond this text.

If you could sit everyday for a week, then you have won the first battle; soldier on.

MEDITATION

This practice I have labeled *attention* sounds suspiciously like *meditation*, and it is. Meditation is exercise. When we engage in meditation practice we occupy our thoughts with a single point of reference, and we engage the body through breathing, but we do not move. When you practice the forms described in this book you will occupy the mind with a single point of reference--the form practice, but the form practice calls for more attention than monitoring your breath. You will have to be attentive to your posture, to the position of your hands and feet, and the sensations of relaxation or tension that the form practice generates in your body. You will have to do all this, while still concentrating on your breathing. This focus on attention is why the internal martial arts are called *moving meditation*.

Notice that I did not put any structure on this meditation practice other than asking you to note the time you sat down, and the time you got up. I did not ask you to seek enlightenment or reach a higher state of existence, nor did I challenge you to sit for 30 or 60 minutes. This is your practice, and the goals you seek are your own.

This book does not burden you with increasing numbers of exercises that you must do daily to grow. Rather, it has many different exercises that you can perform during your daily moment of attention. The idea is to have variety. Variety is the spice of life.

In the Introduction I shared my personal journey and how on at least one occasion I had become disconnected from my practice and how events happened to reconnect me.

Taking time to write down your personal journey and reviewing it for landmarks that were transformational in your life is the only way, I can think of, that you will know yourself. What

I have learned from my journaling practice is that the transformational moments are not what you expected.

You expect the transformational moments to be things like graduating from school, or starting a new job. I find they are more subtle, like the pop of a joint, or the discovery of a new hobby. You do not recognize these new milestones because you are not paying attention.

If you are using a journal with your practice or not, I encourage you to write down some goals for your practice, but do not put a timeframe around them. If you cannot think of any goals, simply write down your reason for practicing Baguazhang (that you chose in the previous section), and review this list before you start to practice each day.

STANDING

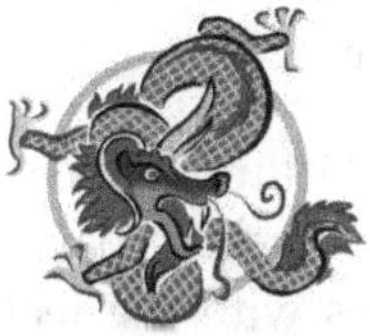

Before you begin the physical exercises in this book, you will stand in Wuji Posture and clear your mind of other thoughts. This is similar to the attention practice from the previous section. Except in your standing practice, you will begin developing awareness of your body.

Remember the story of the egg in the Origins section where "there was nothing but a formless chaos." This is the state of *Wuji*. Before creation there was nothing, no form, no substance, just void and nothingness. All of existence was present at the beginning of time, and this sum-total of existence was aware of itself in its entirety.

While standing in Wuji Posture your mind will probably fit the *formless chaos* definition--racing from thought to thought. Your body will be still, standing upright without moving. You want to stand until your body and mind are *aware of itself in its entirety.*

Some teachers stress low or wide standing postures as a way to develop strong legs. This creates a condition they call *rootedness.* Being firmly rooted means that it will be more difficult to push you over, and you will have more power to push others away. (The Supplemental Exercises to this section illustrate a shortcut for developing strong legs.)

In my opinion, awareness and rootedness are the same thing. Rootedness implies that you are firmly fixed to the ground, like a tree, or a plant with roots seeking deeply into the soil for nourishment. Standing firm, however, is not the way of internal martial arts. It is with a calm heart and mind that you create your roots. The nourishment you seek in standing practice is both the practice of strong mental focus and physical awareness of your body's place in space and time.

Standing practice is boring, but it will improve the function of your martial forms. Standing--for short periods of time--develops attention to your structural alignment and you will use this knowledge for all of your subsequent practice.

There are different versions of the Wuji Posture demonstrated by different martial forms and different teachers have different interpretations. There are Wuji postures with the feet placed next to each other, and postures with the feet placed at shoulder width. Some have the toes angled outward and others point the toes straight ahead.

Before I became more aware of functional body alignment, I accepted the various Wuji postures as all being correct for that system of practice. After the incident with my hip, however, that changed. The Wuji posture of one system, or even one teacher, became a clue to that system's, or teacher's, overall veracity. Bad functional posture (slouched shoulders, hanging head, toes pointed outward, knees rotated inward) was a sign that a teacher, or a system, did not have, or was not practicing, the fundamentals needed to maintain overall health.

Today, we know that the human body is bilateral in all of its joints because anything else would not work. There are two of everything you need to move in an upright posture. Two ankles are supported by two knees that leverage the force of a step and produce the ability to walk. The knees are attached to your torso by two hips that give you the flexibility to reach the ground from above and to change directions at will. Above the hips, two shoulders are attached to two elbows that multiply force and extend your agility into new angles. The two elbows are attached

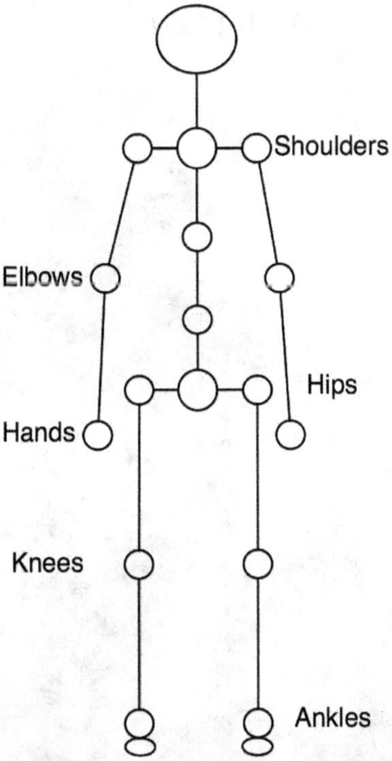

Functional Joints

to two wrists that provide you the finest dexterity. Finally you have two hands filled with equal numbers of fingers that can act in opposition to each other, or in complete harmony.

WUJI POSTURE

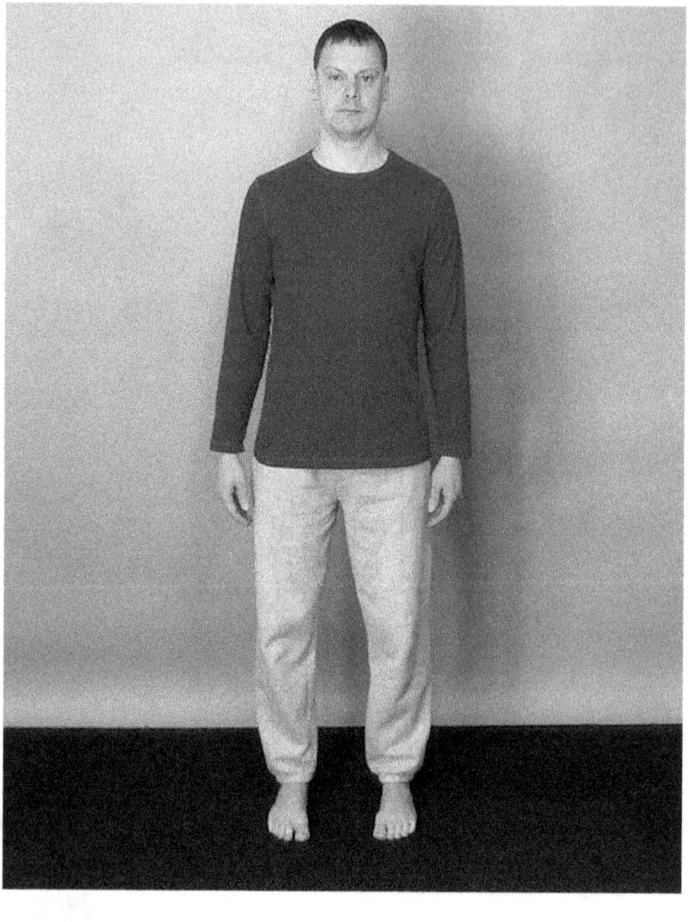

Wuji Posture

Stand up, put your hands at your sides and examine yourself. Is one toe pointing out or one shoulder higher than the other? Does one palm face the front and the other face your side? Your standing posture is a reflection of the disfunction years of inattentiveness has caused. It is time to pay attention to your standing posture, know how your body is functioning today, and take responsibility to create a new milestone for yourself and your ability to stand on your own two feet.

The best way I have found to assume a functional Wuji Posture is to stand with my heels together and feet pointing out so that there is a 90 degree angle between them. Once you have this position turn on your little toes causing the heels to separate from each other and come to rest under your hips. You should have your feet under your hips--that is, they should be hip width apart. The big toe of each foot should be pointing forward or slightly in.

Your knees should be pointing straight ahead and not rounded in or out. You may find that you need to apply some tension along the inside or outside of your thighs to keep the knees pointing forward. As your leg strength improves, this will not be needed.

The weight should fall along the entire foot and balance between both feet. You can create the correct feeling in your feet by grabbing the floor with your toes. Do not curl your toes under, just hug the floor as though you are trying not to slip. This will create a slight arch in the foot that distributes the weight along the functional parts.

Since you have been looking at your toes, you need to straighten your torso up. You can do this by pulling your tail bone in and up, as if you were clenching something between your buttocks. Check the lower back for an excessive curve by running your hand along the lower spine. It should be mostly flat, however, a lower back arch is normal, and you should not trust any instruction that tries to eliminate it.

Next, you need to pull your head up by pretending you have a string attached to the crown of your skull and someone is pulling up on the string. I have even pulled my own hair up from this point just to reinforce the image. The effect should be that the chin tucks in slightly, and there is a flat line from the shoulder blades to the top your head. If have pulled your shoulders back correctly, they will be under your ears.

Finally, tighten the whole posture by really pulling back on the shoulder blades and clenching the buttocks and pushing the hands firmly against the thighs, then relax and stand naturally in this posture.

If your job has you on your feet all day, you are more aware of your posture than you may think. Standing in this posture will reinforce your attention and bring your functional alignments into your awareness.

There is very little that can go wrong by standing in Wuji Posture. Some side effects that you may feel include stiff shoulders and neck (indicating that you need to reinforce your Wuji Posture practice with upper body exercise) tingling in the legs and feet (indicating that you need to walk more) and stiffness in the lower back (indicating that your back is probably holding you up and not your legs). When you feel uncomfortable, walk about for a couple of minutes, then return to Wuji Posture.

The legends say that the old masters would stand in Wuji Posture for hours on end. I recommend standing in Wuji Posture for one to ten minutes, with three to five minutes being ideal. You can mark this time with a clock or by setting a timer, but I prefer to time my practice with my breathing. When you first start to practice your breaths will be shorter but as your practice improves, you will regulate your breathing and your breaths will grow longer. Early on in my practice I determined that I was breathing between 12 and 15 times per minute when I was exercising. I just took the larger number and called that one minute. I figured that as I did a better job of regulating my breathing my standing practice would naturally become longer. Using your breathing as a guide, stand in Wuji Posture for 15 to 45 breaths.

SUPPLEMENTAL EXERCISES

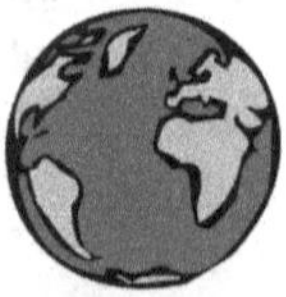

I have collected several exercises to supplement my martial art practice. These are isometric or stretching movements that have improved my general health. I feel that it is important to link the exercises to the traditional forms so you know what is improved by the floor exercise. Therefore, as you progress through this book, please take some time to do the floor exercises as well.

BEAR POSTURE

This posture is designed to just let all the stress of the day go, and I will refer to it often.

Find a chair, bed, foot stool, anything that is about the height of your knees and wide enough for your legs to lie on. In this example, I use a chair.

Lie on your back, with your arms extended at your sides,

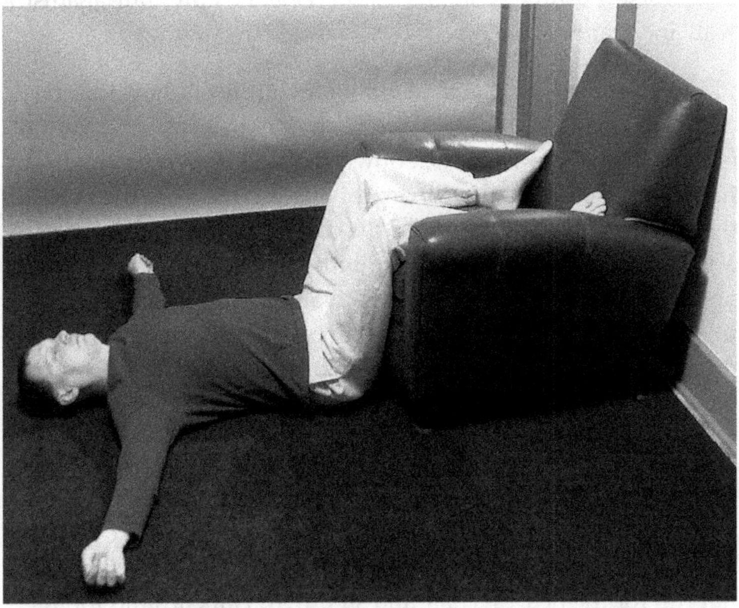

Bear Posture

and put your feet onto the chair. Slide your bottom next to the chair so that you form two 90 degree angles: one from your knees to your thighs, and the second from your thighs to your hips and back. This is a relaxing posture, but it is not doing anything to strengthen your shoulders, hips, legs, or lower back, so no more than 15 minutes at a time.

HORSE POSTURE

Traditional martial art teaching includes a low and wide stance known as *Ma Bu,* or Horse Stance. This stance develops leg strength, or rootedness. As I explained earlier, we are abandoning the wide and deep stances for proper alignment and function. This does not mean, however, that we can abandon leg strength.

We need a posture that can engage our leg muscles in a functional manner without dedicating hours to just standing around. The Horse Posture is similar to the Bear Posture, but against a wall and standing up.

Find a sturdy wall and stand with your heels, buttocks, back, and head against it. Step out from the wall about two-foot-lengths, then slide your back down the wall until your thighs are flat. There should be two 90 degree angles, one from the knees to the thighs, and the other from the thighs to your hips and back. Your feet are flat on the floor with the toes pointing straight ahead. Do not push back into the wall any more than is needed to keep you upright. Lay your hands on your thighs with the palms facing up, and relax the shoulders. (Note that I practice barefoot. You may want to wear some shoes with a good grip to prevent your feet from sliding.)

Hold this position for up to three minutes (45 breaths). It is a challenge. When finished, slide back up the wall and get your feet under you before you stand up. As tempting as it will be, do not run for the nearest chair and sit down. Walk around for a few minutes, paying attention to how your legs feel now that you have reengaged the thighs.

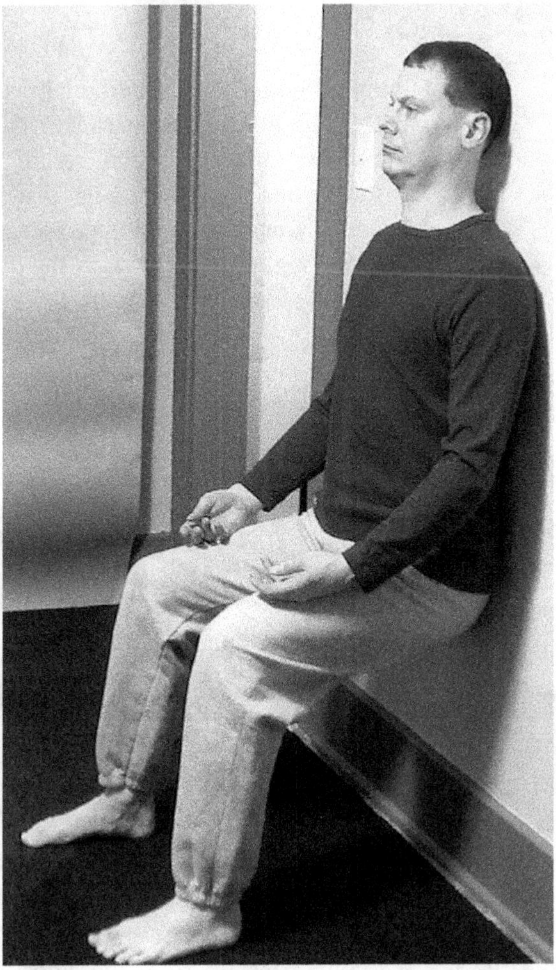

Horse Posture

The old masters were trying to encourage the same result with low and deep horse stances. Standing in any of the postures presented here for an extended time would reengage the leg muscles. Horse Posture is a shortcut that accomplishes the same thing.

HOLDING THE MOON

Holding the Moon is a traditional posture for most Chinese internal martial arts. If you practice Holding the Moon before you are aware of your shoulder and hip alignment, however, you can reinforce bad posture. Therefore, a good way to learn the posture is lying on the floor.

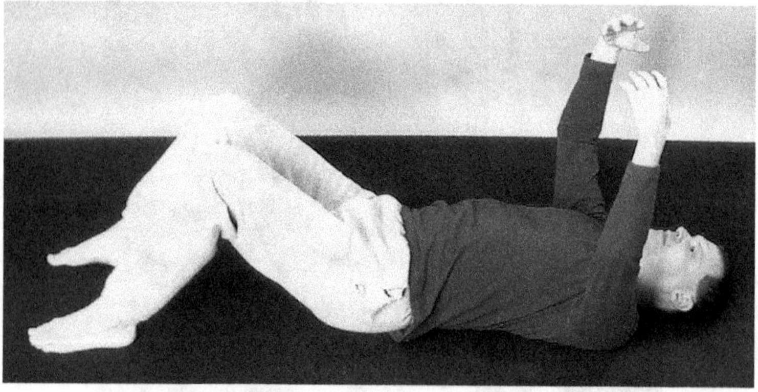

Holding the Moon On the Floor

Lie down on the floor with your feet hip width apart, your arms extended to your sides, and your toes pointing to the ceiling. Pull your feet up by bending your knees until your feet are flat on the floor. Raise your arms up from the sides, bending them at the elbows, until your shoulders start to rise off the floor. Gravity should pull the elbows and hands down so it looks like you are holding a large ball on your chest. Hold this position for up to five minutes.

In this posture, gravity is trying to pull your arms in any number of directions. If you think of gravity as being water, you can imagine that currents are flowing through the water, trying to push your arms down to the floor by dragging them over your head, or by pushing them out to the sides. You are resisting the flow of water, holding your arms up with your hands over your shoulders.

You want to supply just enough resistance in the arms to keep them in the correct position. This idea of providing just enough tension to hold the position is called *sung. Sung* is often translated as relax, but you do not want to relax so much that you become a bowl of jelly. Holding the Moon on the Floor posture is a good way to experience this idea of *sung*. Since the rest of your body is being supported by the floor, you can put your attention on the arms. Try different levels of tension and relaxation in your arm muscles as you breathe deeply. When you find a combination that feels most comfortable, you have achieved *sung*.

The standing version of Holding the Moon Posture is one of those exercises that looks really simple, but can be a serious challenge, especially if your hips and shoulders are weak. Once you are comfortable with the Wuji Posture, you can add Holding the Moon to your standing practice by raising the arms straight out to shoulder height and letting the elbows sink down and away so the palms turn inwards.

When you are in the standing posture, gravity is pulling down on the arms, like they are *sinking* into the water. This *sinking* feeling is called *chen.* Once you become familiar with *sung* and *chen* in your arms, start putting your attention on other parts of your body, and applying these principles. For example, your shoulders should be pulled back, with the shoulder blades under your ears, *relaxed,* and *sinking* to the ground.

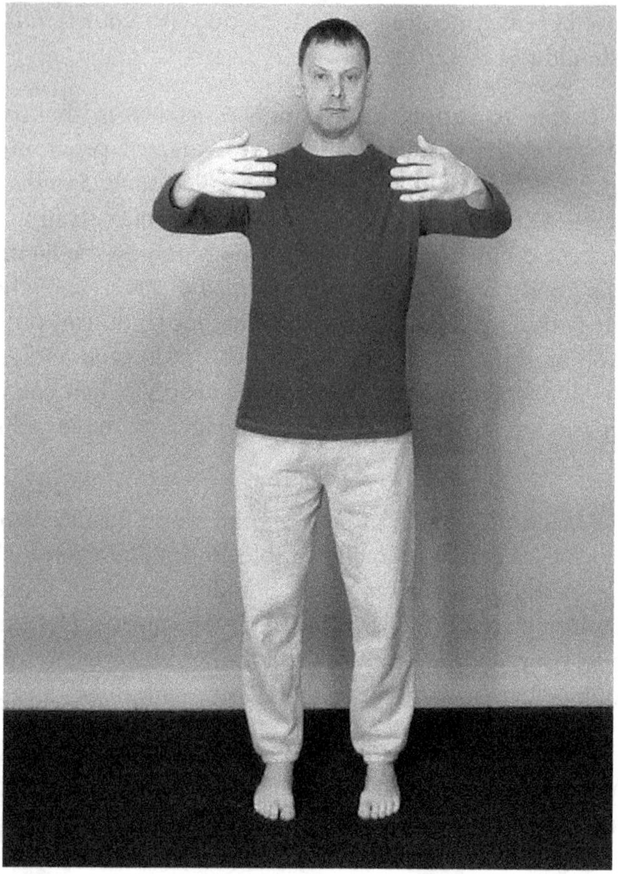

Holding the Moon Posture

SUPPLEMENTAL EXERCISE

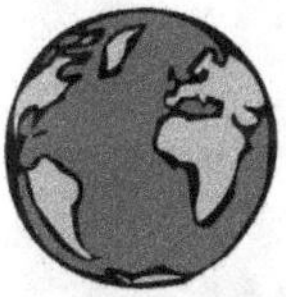

While Standing in Holding the Moon Posture, you will become reacquainted with the muscles of your shoulders. Here are some exercises to engage those muscles and improve your practice.

ARM CIRCLES

One exercise that helps to strengthen and improve the shoulder range of motion is the traditional Arm Circle exercise.

Stand in Wuji Posture with your arms at your sides. Raise your arms with the palms facing to the floor, and pull your shoulder blades back. Circle your arms in the direction of your thumb, forward in this case, but do not make the circles too wide. Your hands should not travel below your ribs, or above your head, when doing Arm Circles. Perform 50 to 100 repetitions in this direction. Try to keep the shoulder blades pulled back through the entire exercise. It helps to look into a mirror when doing this exercise so you can see the range of motion of both arms.

After 50 to 100 repetitions forward, turn your hands over, so the palms are facing up, and perform 50 to 100 repetitions in the other direction.

PUSH UPS

Lie flat on your stomach with your head and nose touching the floor. Place your hands about six inches away from your shoulder blades. The elbows should be pointing straight up to the ceiling. Exhale as you push away from the floor and inhale as

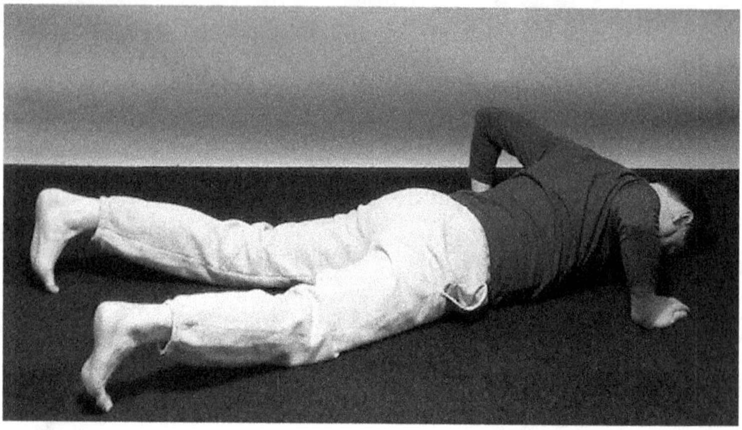

Push Ups - One

you lower back to the floor. A set of 25 Push Ups is a good place to start, and you probably do not need more than that, if you are practicing them daily.

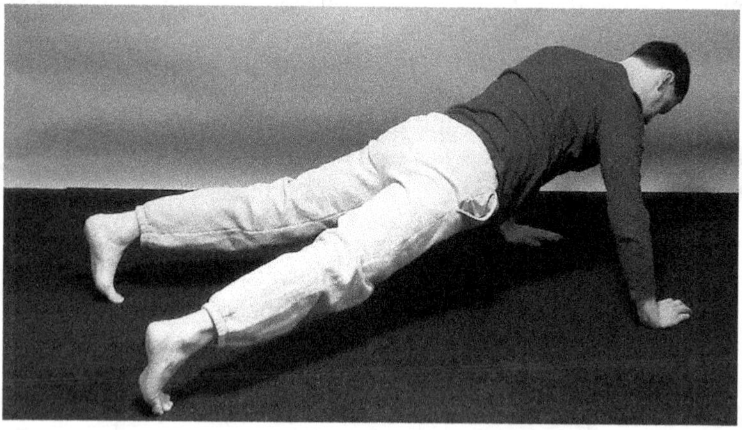

Push Ups - Two

YIN YANG POSTURE

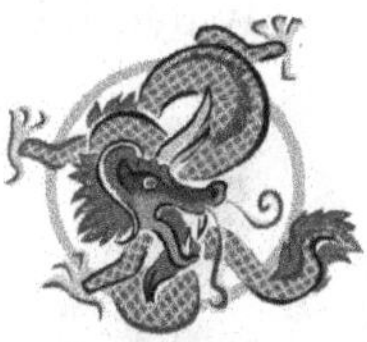

The Yin Yang Posture introduces the idea of movement into your standing practice. By shifting the weight onto one leg and letting the other leg hang empty in space you are training the body how it will feel to move without moving. This idea of stillness and motion coexisting relates to the Yin and Yang theory. The Yin Yang Posture lets you practice this mutual coexistence without moving. Later, you will practice this mutual coexistence while moving.

Remember that the concept of Yin and Yang is as ancient as Chinese philosophy. The origin story said that there was a primordial chaos--Wuji--out of which an egg was born. When the egg split the heavy yolk sank to become the Earth--Yin--while the light egg white rose to become the Heavens--Yang.

Yin and Yang are represented by two lines. Yang is a solid line that represents brightness, lightness, masculinity, and the tendency to move upwards. Yin is a broken line that represents darkness, heaviness, femininity, and the tendency to move downwards.

When standing in the Yin Yang Posture you can imagine that the solid leg is heavy and downward seeking--Yin. While the open leg is light and floating upwards--Yang. Likewise, you can imagine that the solid leg is active and represents the solid Yang line, while the open leg is passive and represents the broken Yin line. I will call the solid leg the Yin leg, and the open leg the Yang leg.

No one thing is completely Yin or completely Yang; each contains the seed of its opposite. For example, winter eventually turns into summer. After you stand in Yin Yang posture on the left side, you change positions and the Yin leg will become Yang, and *vice-versa*.

Any Yin or Yang aspect can be further subdivided into Yin and Yang. For example, temperature can be seen as either hot (Yang) or cold (Yin). However, hot can be further divided into

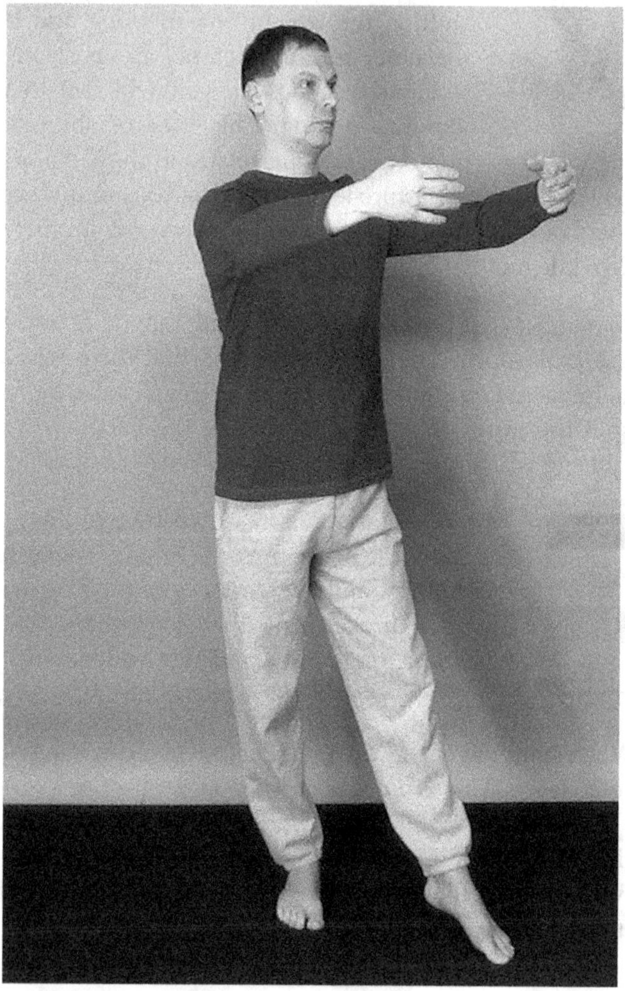

Yin Yang Posture

warm or burning; cold into cool or icy. Within each spectrum, there is a smaller spectrum. As you stand in Yin Yang posture, you will find that the Yang leg begins to feel heavy--Yin qualities within the Yang leg. Likewise, the Yin leg may begin to tingle or even twitch--Yang qualities within the Yin leg.

To assume the Yin Yang left posture, stand in Holding the Moon Posture and then turn the left heel to touch the ankle of the right foot. Kick out with the left foot and let the big toe just touch the floor. The alignments that you practiced in Wuji Posture remain the same, except the left knee and foot is now pointing 45 degrees to the left. The torso turns naturally with the leg.

This is another chance to remind you of the four keys to good internal martial art posture. The first is the tucking in of the chin and raising of the back of the head. The second is the pulling up of the pelvis without eliminating the lower back arch; in other words, do not slouch forward or bend backward. The third is to keep the knees open and feel as though you are sinking into the floor. After you have assumed the Yin Yang Posture, run a quick scan of your body and determine if those three keys are still in place. Then breathe deeply and practice *sung*--the fourth key.

In the Yin Yang Posture there should be a continuous line from the heel to the shoulder of the supporting leg, and a continuous line from the toe to the shoulder of the open leg. Focus on maintaining these alignments, as you breathe and relax.

Stand in left Yin Yang Posture for three minutes (45 breaths) before changing to right Yin Yang Posture.

SUPPLEMENTAL EXERCISE

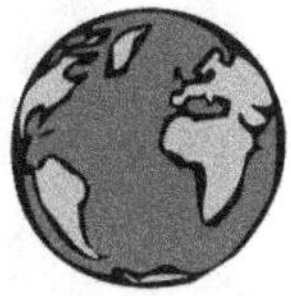

There are some crazy exercises to open the hips and regain flexibility in the pelvic girdle. Some of them involve a partner pushing or pulling legs to ever wider angles. Those just seem painful to me, and I should know, because I have tried some of them in the past. Here is an exercise that you can do lying on your stomach and back that will open and relax the hip joints without having to become a contortionist.

BUTTERFLY

Lie on your stomach with you hands above your head. The alignment of the body should be as we discussed in the Wuji Posture, but lying flat on the floor. Turn your head to the left so the right cheek and ear are against the floor. Breathe deeply and slowly. Now pull your left leg up so the foot is at the height of the right knee, and the left knee is level with the hip. The left

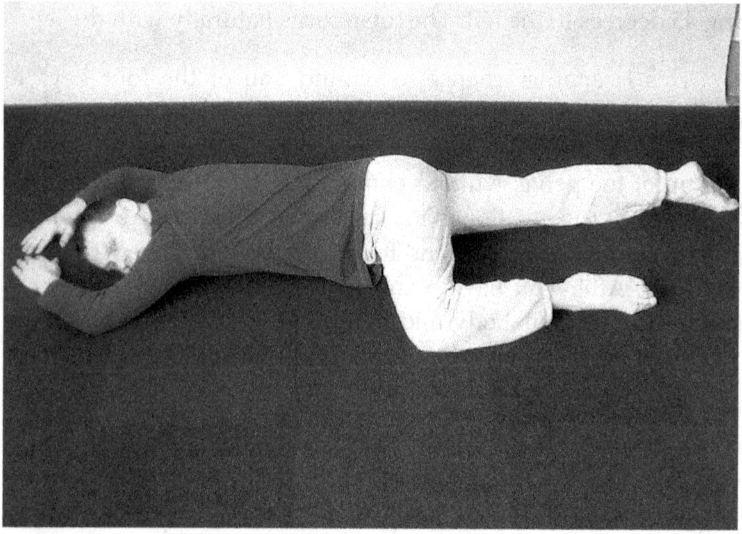

Butterfly - Front

foot is below the left hip. If you cannot get the foot to knee height without experiencing some discomfort, then stop where it starts to hurt. Hold this position for a minute before straightening the left leg

To repeat on the right side, turn your head to the right so the left cheek and ear are against the floor and then raise the right leg. Hold this position for a minute.

Repeat the entire exercise up to three times before rolling onto your back.

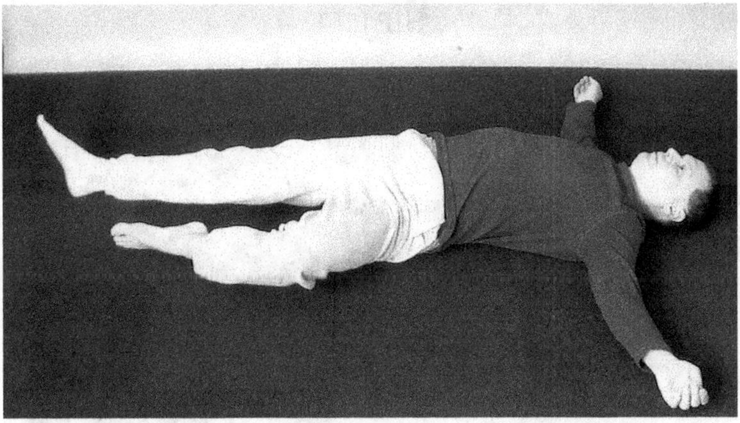

Butterfly - Back

Lie on your back in Wuji Posture with the toes pointing to the ceiling. Extend your arms out to the side as you did in Bear Posture. Look at the ceiling and bend your left knee so that the left foot rises to the height of the right knee. Let the knee fall outward and the hip open up as you raise the foot. The sole of the left foot points to the right leg. Hold for a minute before straightening the leg and repeating on the right side.

HIP LIFT

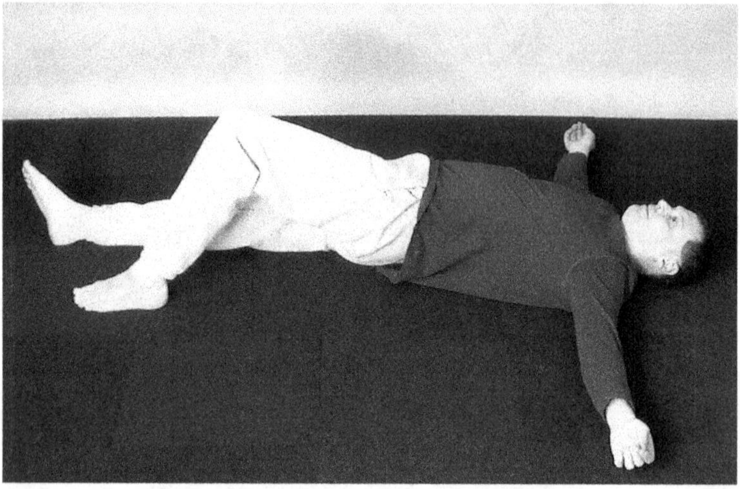

Hip Lift

Lie on your back in proper Wuji Posture alignment, but extend your arms to the sides with your palms facing up. Pull the left foot up so it is opposite the right knee. Keep the sole of the left foot flat on the floor. Push down through the left foot so the left hip and side rise off the floor. This will cause you to twist to the right, but let your right shoulder and arm stop you from rolling over. Hold the position for one to three minutes (15 to 45 breaths).

When you are finished straighten the left leg and repeat the exercise on the right side.

The key to doing this exercise correctly is keeping the knee of the bent leg pointing straight up.

TRINITY POSTURE

San Ti Shi, or the Three Body Posture combines the lessons of Wuji and Yin Yang Posture and integrates martial intent. In this posture, the body is divided into three sections that are further divided into three more sections. The primary division is the head, the hands, and the feet. The head section is divided into the head, the spine and the waist. The hands section is divided into the hands, the elbows, and the shoulders. The feet section is divided into the feet, the knees, and the hips.

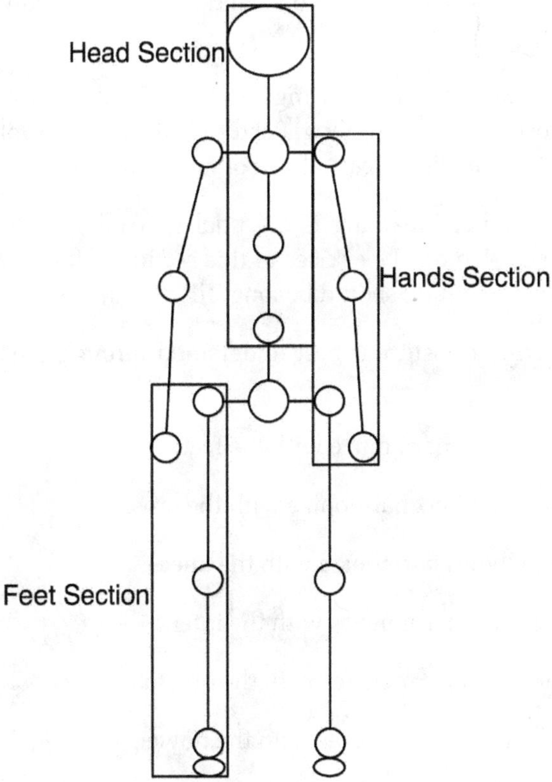

The "Three Bodies" of Trinity Posture

In the diagram, notice how each of the primary sections are linked through the shoulders and hips.

All martial arts have some form of the Trinity Posture; it is also called the *on-guard* stance. The basics are always the same, however: one leg back with more weight on it, the front leg able to move quickly into another position. One hand back and on-guard from incoming attacks, with the other hand stretched forward, feeling out the opponent.

Teachers of the Xingyiquan martial art often ask their students to stand in Trinity Posture for hours before any movements are practiced. In some schools the form is not even discussed. The teachers just let you stand around until you figure it out.

If you have been practicing the Wuji Posture, Holding the Moon Posture, and Yin Yang Posture with their supplemental exercises you are light years ahead of most students.

Since proper breathing is essential to Trinity Posture practice, the supplemental exercises to this section will cover breathing. Proper breathing should be long, silent, and deep.

The Trinity Posture is best understood through the Six Harmonies:

- The hands harmonize with the feet.
- The shoulders harmonize with the hips.
- The elbows harmonize with the knees.
- The heart harmonizes with the intent.
- The intent harmonizes with the breath.
- The breath harmonizes with the power.

These harmonies are the cornerstone of Xingyiquan practice, and they reveal the *secret* training of the internal martial artist.

I have divided them into their *external* and *internal* components.

THE EXTERNAL HARMONIES

As you learned in the Wuji Posture lesson, the human body is bilateral and level in both the horizontal and vertical planes--except for those cases where some trauma has injured the body. The easiest way to see this, is to look at the major joints that form most of our structure and provide the means for locomotion both horizontally and vertically.

When standing or walking, take a few minutes to find this functional alignment in your posture before you begin practice. Become aware of how the whole body is a unified machine. Your toes are not separate from your shoulders, but connected in a long and continuous webbing of muscles, ligaments, nerves, and blood vessels.

The hands harmonize with the feet

Any movement of the hand must be accompanied by an appropriate movement of the foot. The slightest step or push is generated from the feet, transmitted through the legs into the torso and through the shoulders to finally be expressed in the hands.

The shoulders harmonize with the hips

Aligning shoulder movement with hip movement turns the torso slightly from the line of attack. This subtle turn can be the difference between life and death in a fight. More important, it unifies the power of the legs with the arms.

The elbows harmonize with the knees

This harmony is more about protecting the body, than functional alignment. The elbows are often the torso's only defense from a strike. In the martial art of Xingyiquan this function is emphasized by the statement: "The elbows do not leave the ribs, the hands do not leave the heart." Harmonizing the elbows with the knees means that you will not overextend the arms and legs. It also implies that the elbows must drop--or sink--downward despite the position of the hands.

Do not assume that the external harmonies mean that the right side of the body moves or functions in unison, and then the left side. The left foot and right hand can act in harmony. This is illustrated by the natural walking, or gait, pattern of the left leg and foot extending forward while the right arm and hand pull back, then the right leg and foot extending forward while the left arm and hand pull back.

This unity of body, however, cannot be accomplished with physical action alone. It requires attention, and intention. The internal trinity is the recipe for focusing on the task of unification.

THE INTERNAL HARMONIES

The heart harmonizes with the intent

A student of meditation will understand that there is more than one mind in the human body. Some meditation schools describe three minds, the gut, the heart and the one in the head. Others, have two; the heart and the one in the head (the emotional and the rational). The heart mind is where your anger, fear, joy, and sorrow come from. This is the mind in your chest and gut. The rational mind is where logic, thinking, mathematics, and language come from. This is the mind in your head. The heart harmonizing with the intent means that the emotional mind and the rational mind act together.

The idea that you would not engage in practice without first harmonizing the emotional and rational minds recalls the Buddhist Eightfold Path and the Daoist concept of Wu Wei.

Before you engage in a fight, or martial training, you need to consider what your intentions are. Do you really mean to hurt someone? Is fighting the right action? If engaging in combat is the right response then you need to be of one mind about the decision. There are legends of martial art masters hair standing on end and eyes focusing such violence that their challengers surrendered. If there is any doubt between the rational mind and the heart mind, then fighting is not the answer. Back down, apologize, and walk away.

The intent harmonizes with the breath

When you are of one mind, engage it in your practice with your breath. One breath in, one breath out, completes one cycle. Breathing in will coordinate with opening movements, defending, and expanding. Breathing out will coordinate with closing movements, attacking, and sealing up. No movement is executed without the breath.

The breath harmonizes with the power.

As you breathe in the power is collected; as you breathe out the power is expressed. No movement happens without the breath; it is the engine of your practice.

Understanding the Six Harmonies is the purpose of practice. Practice will create experiences that bring further understanding. Understanding will inspire new questions that can only be answered with more practice.

STANDING IN TRINITY POSTURE

Assume the Yin Yang left posture, with the left foot empty and the right foot holding your weight. Bend the right knee down so you can reach forward with the heel of your left foot and place it where your toes were in the Yin Yang posture.

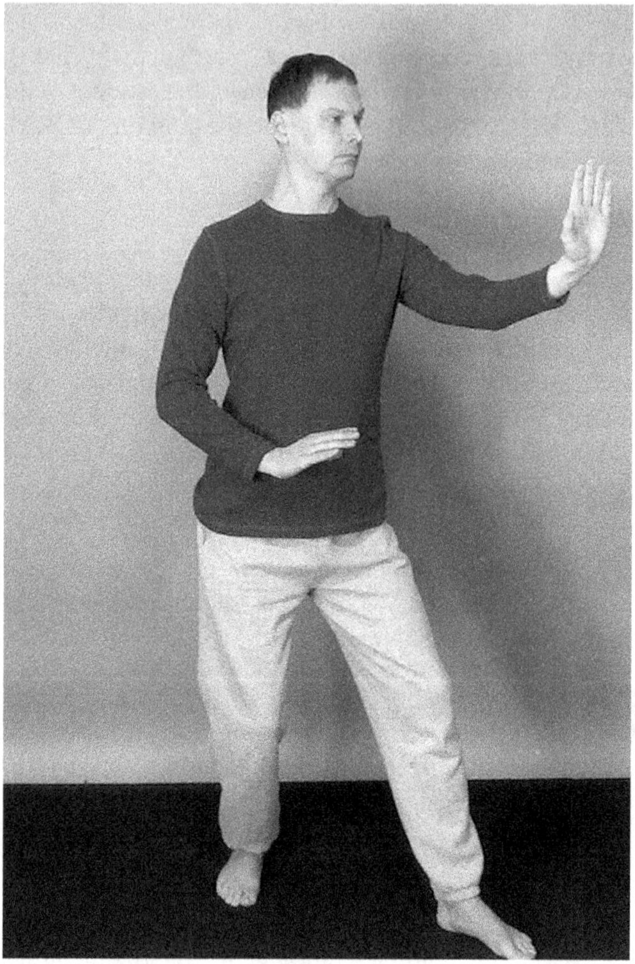

Trinity Posture - Left

Lower the right hand so it fits under the rib cage on your right side. The thumb can be as far forward as the belly button, or as far back as the kidney. The left hand remains in place, but the palm turns to face away from you, as if you are pushing against something.

Now that you are in the posture, breathe deeply and focus your gaze between the thumb and forefinger of the left hand (this is called the *tiger's mouth*). As you breathe in, imagine that an object in the distance is being pulled to you, when you breathe out, imagine that the object is being pushed away.

Count the breaths, and check your posture every 15 breaths. Ensure that you have not slumped down, that your hands are in the correct position, that your chin is tucked in, the back of the head is raised, and that you have not leaned to the left or right.

After three to five minutes in the left facing Trinity Posture, re-center to the Wuji Posture and then stand in the right facing Trinity Posture for three to five minutes.

SUPPLEMENTAL EXERCISE

DEEP BREATHING

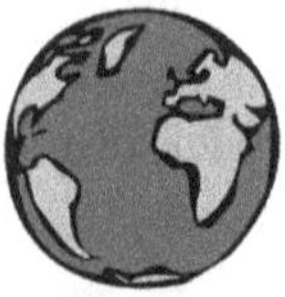

Until you can breathe deeply and slowly it will be impossible for you to coordinate the internal and external harmonies into a unified practice.

A good way to start breath practice is in the Bear Posture. Instead of holding your hands out to your sides, put the left hand on your lower abdomen and the right hand on your chest.

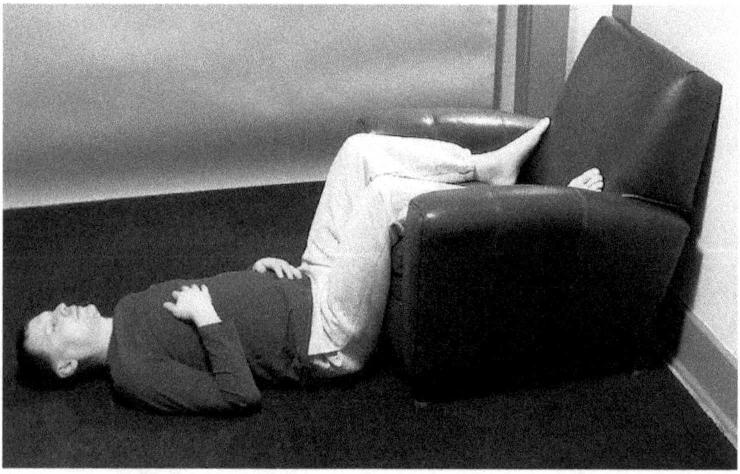

Deep Breathing in Bear Posture

Breathe in through your nose. Take a very deep breath bringing in as much air as possible. As you breathe in raise the lower abdomen up as if you are inflating a balloon. Hold your breath long enough to try the next step.

Push down on the lower abdomen with the left hand. As you push down with the hand pull the abdomen down from inside as well. The breath should feel as though it is moving up and into the chest. Then push the breath back down into the abdomen with the right hand, and allow the abdomen to expand. Repeat this transfer three times before letting the air out in a long smooth flow through your nose.

Take a few moments and then repeat the exercise up to five times. When breathing in and out, doing so silently will lengthen the breath and focus your attention.

This exercise focuses entirely on the breath and how it moves in your body. Become aware of how a full deep breath feels. Be attentive to the pressure the air creates. When performing martial forms you will breathe in as you open and breathe out as you close. The old masters said that adding breath to the movement generated power. When performing the exercise consider how the internal pressure of your breath being released could generate added force in a push.

THE BELLOWS

Breathing in is Yin, breathing out is Yang. When performing the martial forms, breathing in is associated with defensive movements, while breathing out is associated with offensive movements. This exercise coordinates breathing with movement

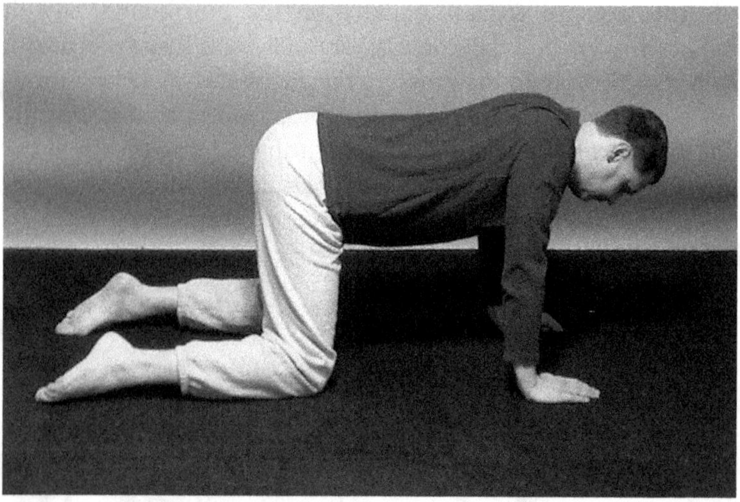

The Bellows -- One

while exercising the spine, shoulders, and hips.

Start on your hands and knees, with the hands directly under the shoulders, and the knees directly under the hips. The back is relaxed, while the shoulders are pushed back (upwards) by the weight of the body.

Breathe in as you arch your back and roll your shoulders forward (down). Breath out as you return to the original position. Perform 25 repetitions with deep long breaths acting as the engine to your bellows.

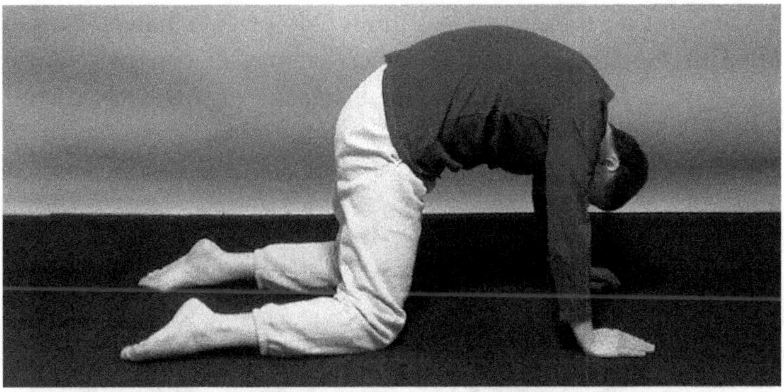

The Bellows -- Two

FINGER EXERCISE

You use our hands all day, yet pay little attention to what they are doing. Studies that map parts of the human body to a brain function draw pictures of the body that represent the relative size of each body part to brain function. These pictures show the hands huge compared to the rest of the body, with one hand being larger than the other.

Bringing your hands into your conscious awareness is the point of this exercise.

Lie down in the Bear Posture and close your eyes, raise your hands up so they are supported by the elbows lying flat on the floor. Close your eyes and slide the fingers of both hands together, letting them interlock in a natural position. Now, move the hands back and forth so the fingers of each hand are gliding against each other. Be attentive to how this feels.

Take the forefinger of one hand and rub it along each finger of the other hand. Repeat with the opposite hand.

Rub the fingers of one hand along the palm and back of the other. Repeat with the other hand.

As you do these exercises think only of your hands. Do not let your thoughts wander to other feelings or concerns of the day. If your thoughts do wander, bring your focus back to your hands.

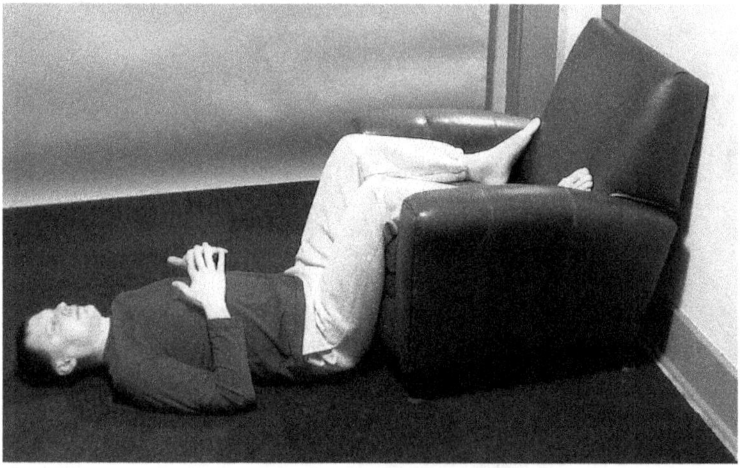

Finger Exercise in Bear Posture

Did you notice that you used your primary hand to start the forefinger exercise? Try the exercise again but start with your secondary hand. Is it harder or easier to remain focused on your hands?

The purpose of this exercise is to become aware of both hands. It is very much like meditation, but you have a physical activity that is the focus of your attention, not unlike martial art practice.

WALKING THE CIRCLE

By taking your standing practice from Wuji Posture through Trinity Posture, with the supplemental exercises, you are well on your way to understanding the whole body connection that makes practicing internal martial arts worthwhile. For Baguazhang practice the next critical component is walking.

WALKING

Walking is a great exercise. The American Heart Association web site lists benefits such as: reduced heart rate, lower blood pressure, improved circulation, and reducing the effects of, or even eliminating, diabetes. Many of the same health benefits attributed to a regular walk are also made about the practice of Taijiquan, Baguazhang, and many other martial styles.

Some added benefits of walking and internal martial art practice, include: improved appetite, weight loss, improved muscle tone, and stronger bones. The American Heart Association and martial art masters also agree that a regular exercise program will reduce the chance of falling, or getting injured by a fall, in your later years. Wouldn't it be great if you could combine martial art practice with the simple act of walking? Well, you can; Baguazhang is a martial art dedicated to walking.

Eight Trigram Palm, or Baguazhang, is the youngest of the Chinese internal martial arts, with much of its growth happening at the beginning of the last century. Despite its newness, it has spread worldwide and is one of the most popularly practiced martial arts.

The basic practice of Baguazhang is easy; you hold fixed postures--from traditional standing practice--while walking in a circle. Walking in a circle forces you to practice a unique toe-in and toe-out step that is crucial to escaping, entering and defeating an opponent. For the Baguazhang martial artist, standing is good, but walking is better.

Baguazhang trains both stillness and movement with the circle walking practice. The beginner learns how to walk, and change directions on the circle while developing leg strength and flexibility in the torso. For anyone who has not suffered a serious misfortune, leg strength is a key to good posture and health.

The mobility gained from circle walking practice gives you an advantage for self-defense. You will learn to change foot and hand positions while moving. This skill to keep moving while defending yourself improves your chance of getting to safety.

Walking in Baguazhang is different from an ordinary stroll. Since you are walking in a circle you are not distracted by your surroundings, allowing you to achieve a meditative state.

The fixed upper body postures stretch and strengthen the torso, and add variety to your practice. You can learn an endless number of ways to change the fixed postures as you change directions on the circle so your practice will not become boring or stagnant.

THE CIRCLE

Before you begin circle walking practice, you need a circle to walk around. As you become comfortable with the stepping pattern needed for good practice, you will not need a visual cue, but it is helpful for beginners. The easiest method is to put an object down and declare that the center of your circle. You could use a coat rack, a tall box, a shoe, anything that helps you find the center to your circle.

I have hung a plant hook in the center of my practice area, and when I am practicing I hang an extendable painter's pole from it. The pole creates a visual reference for my practice, and hides away easily.

Outside, you can create a circle with some sidewalk chalk, marking the edge of a circle on your driveway or patio. If you have access to a gym with a basketball court, you will find that the circle in the middle of the court is a good place to walk about.

The circle needs to be large enough that you are comfortable walking around it. A small circle can cause you to strain your knees or become dizzy quickly. Advanced students walk a circle in eight or ten steps. Beginners should start with a circle two or three times that size.

SUPPLEMENTAL EXERCISE

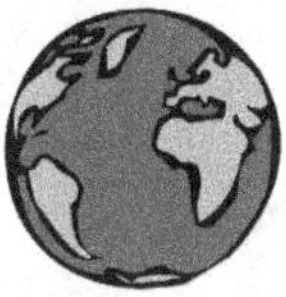

Here are three stretches to do before you walk.

BRIDGE

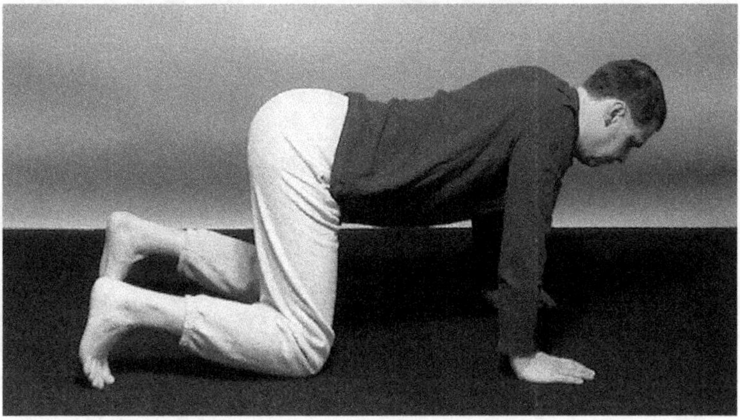

Bridge -- One

The bridge is from a classic pose in Yoga. Start on your hands and knees with the hands beneath the shoulders and the knees beneath the hips.

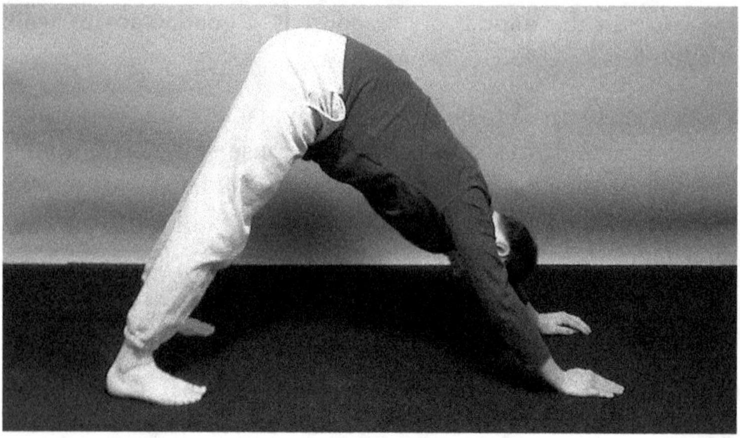

Bridge -- Two

Curl your toes under and then push up through your hands until your feet are flat on the floor. Hold the position for one to three minutes.

HURDLER'S STRETCH

This is one of my favorite stretches. Start on your hands and knees as in the Bridge, but put the left foot in front of the right knee, with the heel touching the knee.

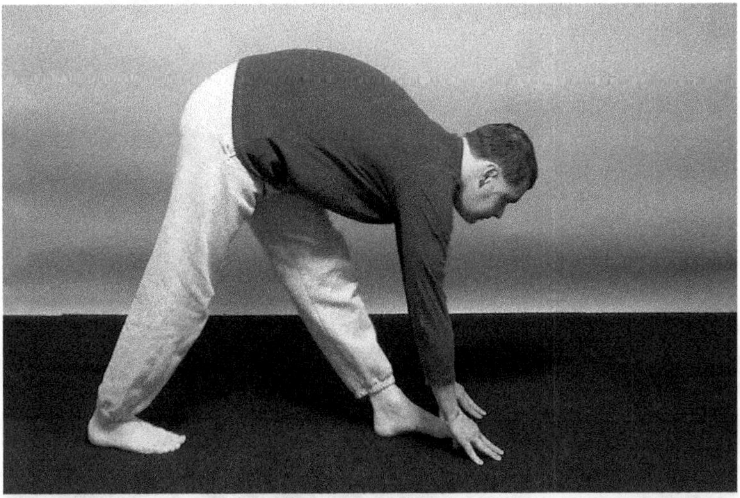

Hurdler's Stretch

Stand up with both feet on the same line and pressing through your fingers. Hold the position for one to three minutes. Not everyone can perform this stretch with their hands on the floor. If you cannot bend this far over, you can supplement the stretch with a chair or stool.

Repeat with the right foot in front of the left knee.

FORWARD BEND

This one may make your hips pop; it is great after sitting too long.

Start from a standing position with your feet spread apart as far as is comfortable.

Forward Bend

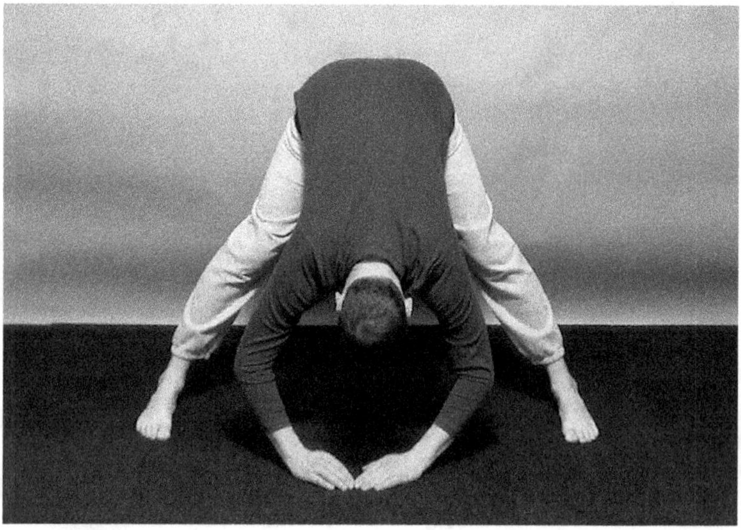

Bend over and put your hands flat on the floor. Again, not everyone can bend this far, and you are welcome to use a chair or stool to supplement the exercise.

Hold the position for one to three minutes.

WUJI WALKING

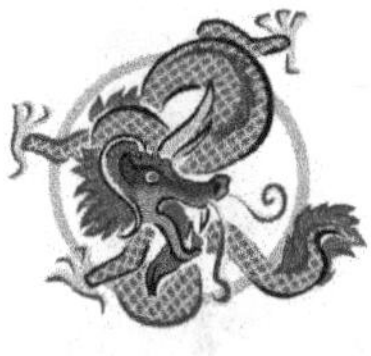

Walking in the Wuji Posture limits your focus to two items: proper body alignment, and walking on the edge of the circle. When you are comfortable moving around the circle in the Wuji Posture, you can progress to the remaining postures.

For beginners, I recommend walking a large circle in the Wuji Posture for more than 10 minutes a day. After a week of daily practice you should make your circle smaller until you can walk a complete circle in eight to ten steps. When you are comfortable walking that size of circle for an extended period, you can progress to more complex postures.

NATURAL WALKING

Stand on the edge of your circle in Wuji Posture facing in a counterclockwise direction. Take eight breaths and become aware of your body alignment. Bend the knees slightly and maintain this bend as you walk. Step forward with the left foot by kicking the left foot out from the knee, and landing the foot on its heel. (For now, use a normal heel-to-toe gait, I will share two alternate forms of walking in the next section.)

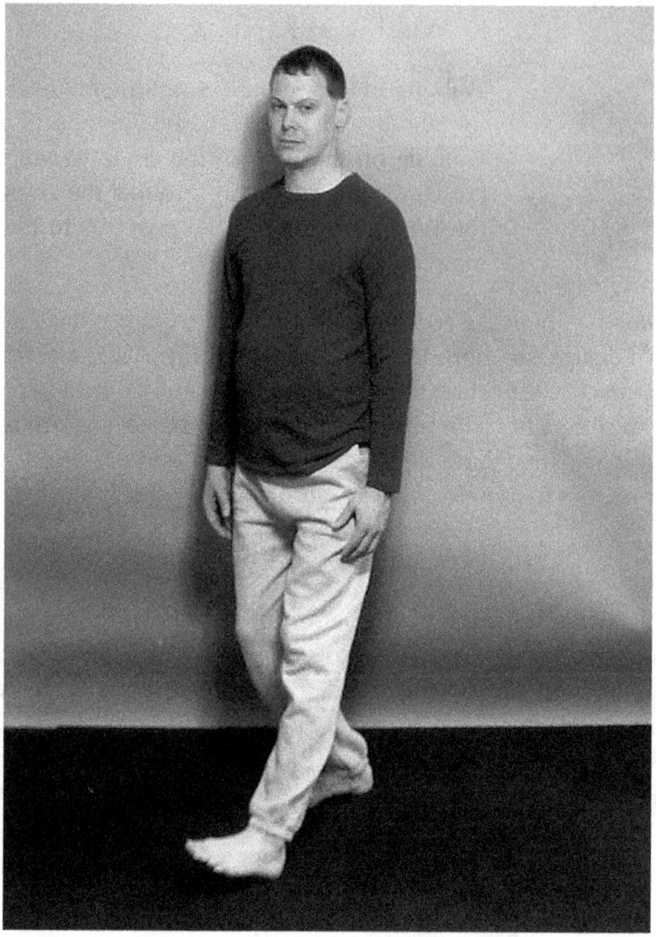

The first step in Wuji Walking

Put the left foot down so it is flat on the floor, and grab the

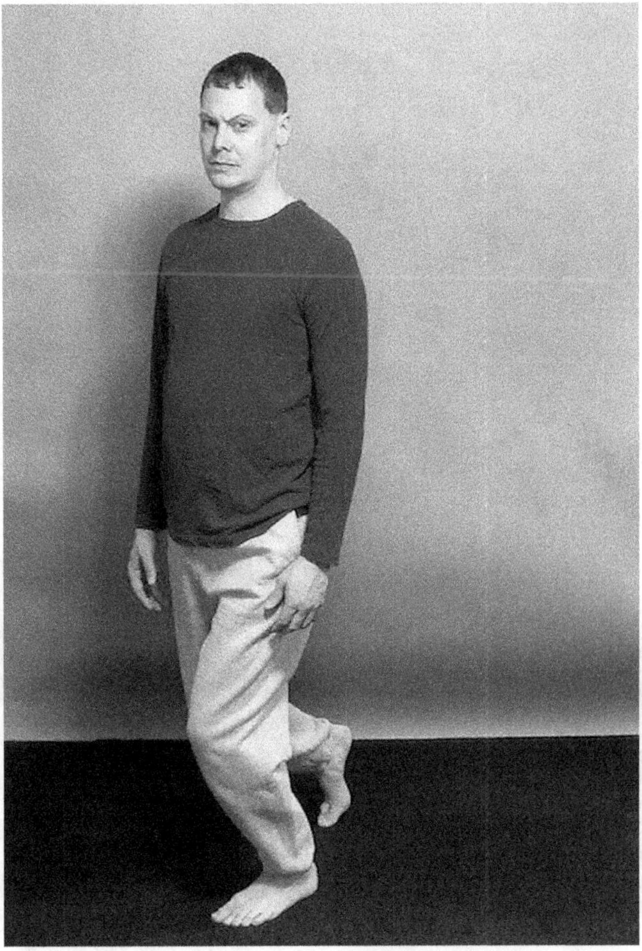

Weight transfer in Wuji Walking

floor slightly with your toes. After the foot is flat on the floor, shift your weight forward onto the left foot and lift the heel of the right foot off the floor.

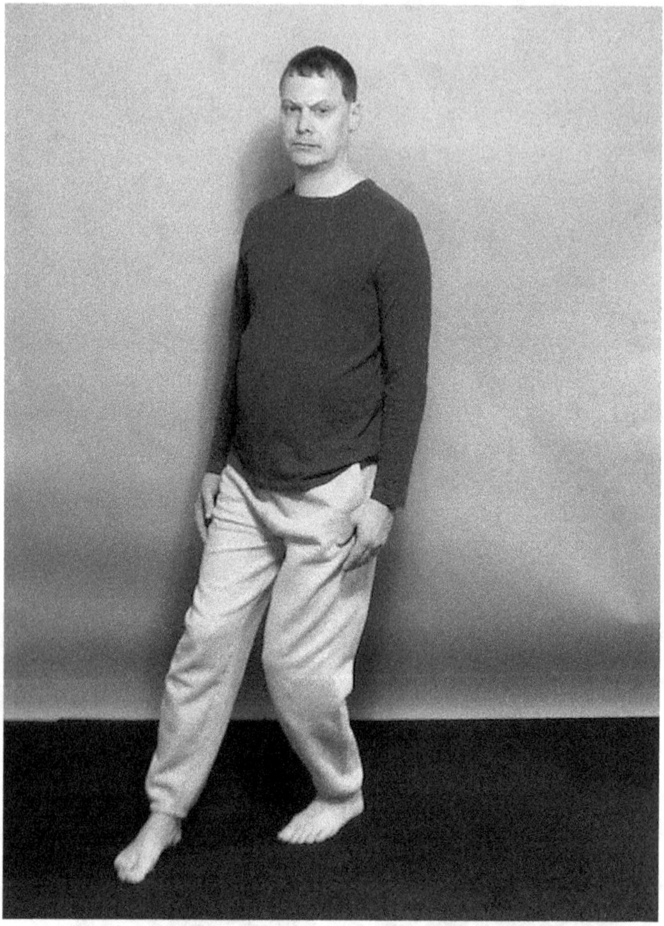

Forming the circle with the right foot

Step up with the right foot, and turn it in slightly so you are walking on the edge of the circle. This slight toe-in step with the outside foot forms the circle. How far you turn the foot into the center of the circle will determine how large a circle you are walking.

Land the right foot on its heel and gradually put it down, grabbing the floor slightly with your toes. Shift your weight onto the right foot as you raise the heel of the left foot. Swing the left foot next to the right and place it in front of the right along the line of the circle. Repeat this stepping pattern over and over until you have completed one circuit.

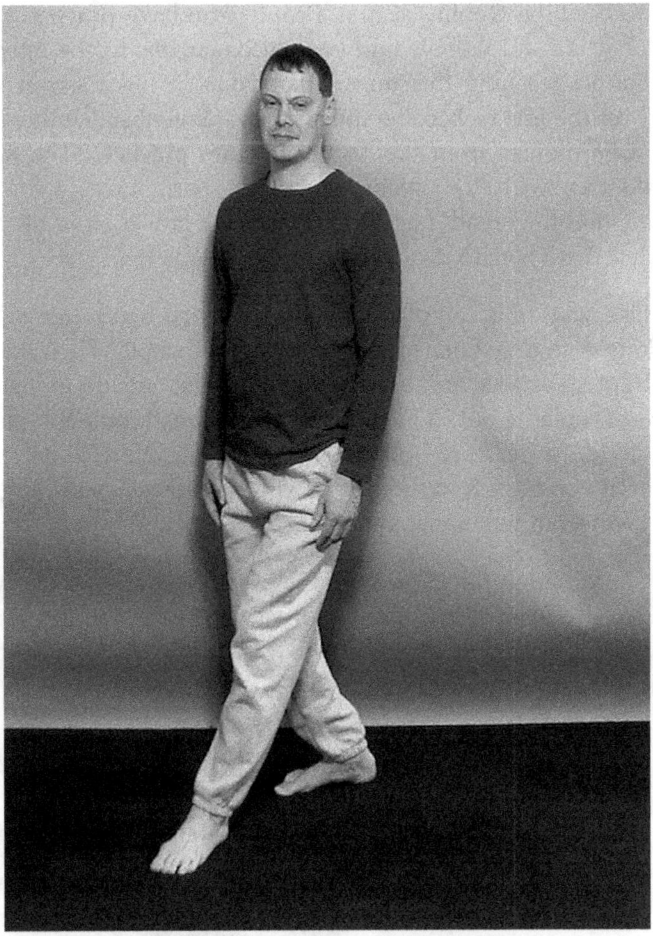

Walking the circle with Scissor Step

As you walk, pay attention to your Wuji Posture, your weight transfer between the feet as you step forward, and keeping your knees bent. Imagine that your legs are the blades of scissors, cutting a piece of paper as you walk. The steps are fairly small, not extending beyond the width of your shoulders. If you are keeping your steps within shoulder width, your knees may rub slightly as you walk, thus reinforcing the *Scissor Step* image.

You will be wobbly at first. People who have practiced this art for years still wobble and sway occasionally. In the internal martial art teaching this means that your Qi has risen. If you sway off the line or become unbalanced, remember the three internal harmonies from the Trinity Posture practice. (The heart harmonizes with the intent, the intent harmonizes with the breath, and the breath harmonizes with the power.) You need to practice them here to avoid being off balance.

One way to accomplish the three internal harmonies while walking is to time your breathing with your steps. When the inside foot steps forward, breathe in; when the outside foot steps forward, breathe out. (One breath in, one breath out, completes one cycle.) If you are still off balance, then make your circle larger. If you have to walk around your entire back yard or gym that is fine, but remember to walk in Wuji Posture.

Coordinating the steps with the breath also means that you will have to walk slowly. Walk at least three circles in this direction before changing directions to walk clockwise around the circle.

SIMPLE CHANGE

The challenge of learning martial forms is practicing the beneficial, boring, movements that train real skill, over the flowery movements that make you look and feel like a superhero. Practicing a few things with purpose is better than practicing many things and losing focus. All martial schools have practice methods that stress a few repeated postures, but such practice is often ignored for the longer, more energetic looking sequences.

Later in this book I will give you an alphabet of directional changes that, if you practice diligently, you can string together to impress your friends with your martial prowess. For now, however, I need you to focus on the footwork and conduct a Simple Change of direction.

With the left foot forward swing the right leg in a tight arc. Land the entire foot on the floor with the toes pointing to the toes of the left foot. Your weight is now equal between both feet, and it should feel like standing in Wuji Posture, except that your toes and knees are pointing towards each other.

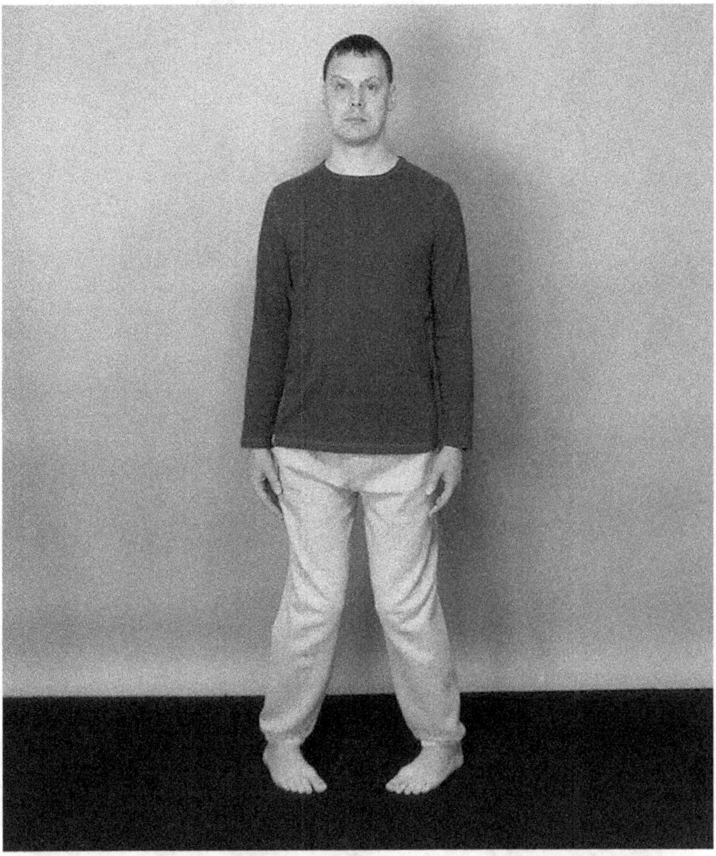

Simple Change - toe-in

If this step was a little small, your knees may be touching. If your knees are touching, slide the right foot out slightly so they separate. Your heels should be about hip width apart.

Take eight breaths and get a feel for this posture before continuing.

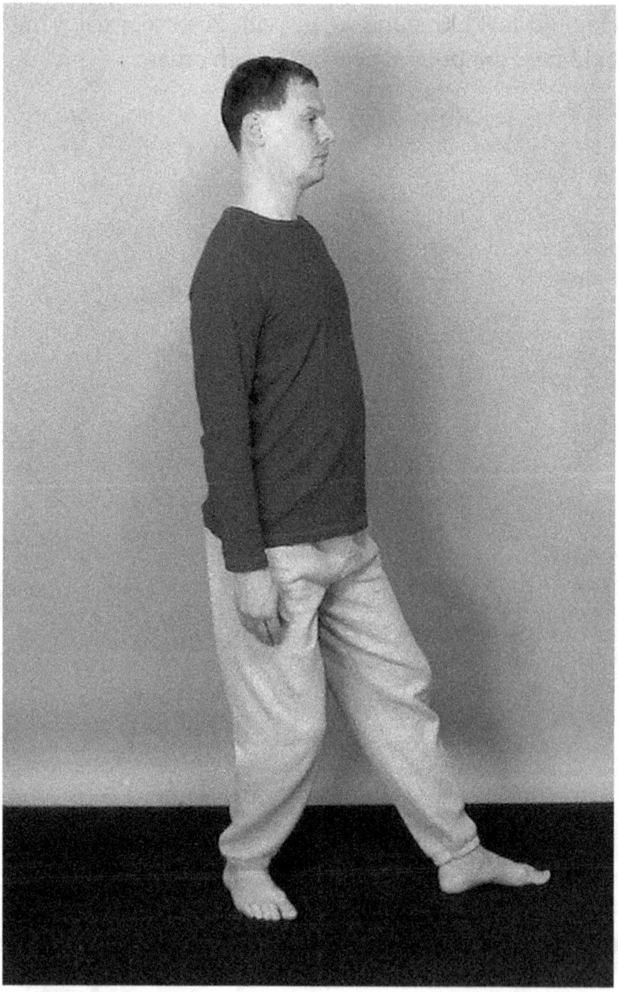

Simple Change - toe-out

Shift your weight onto the right foot and swing the left foot out in an arc, landing it flatly in the same position you used for Yin Yang Posture.

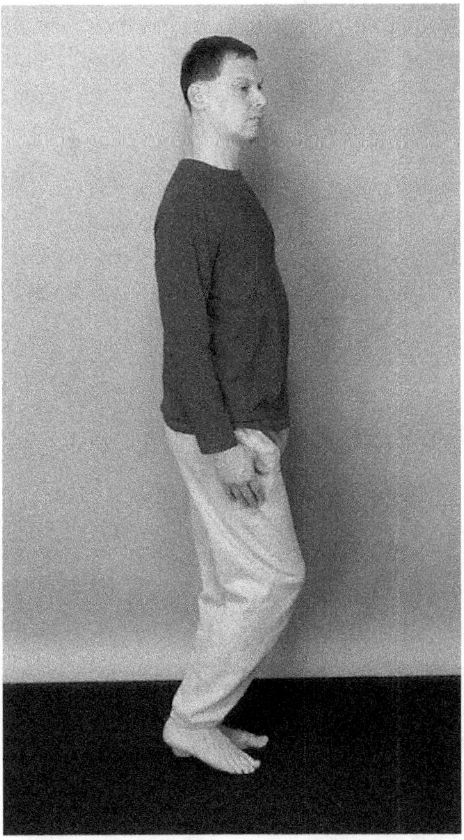

Simple Change - Sweeping Step

Step up slightly with the left foot, landing it on its heel. This is similar to the step you took when you were moving from Yin Yang Posture to Trinity Posture in the Trinity Posture standing exercise. This is called *stealing a step,* and it is a crucial component, do not ignore it.

Continue by bringing the right foot next to the left foot. Stop momentarily with the right foot flat and just off the floor next to the left foot. After this slight pause, sweep the foot forward in a slight arc to begin walking in the clockwise direction. The pause of the right foot next to the left is called a *chicken step.* While the half-arc sweep of the foot after the pause is called a *sweeping step.* Throughout the remainder of this book, I will refer to this entire movement as the Sweeping Step.

Walk at least three circles in the clockwise direction before turning and walking in the counterclockwise direction. When you are ready to stop, simply find a point on the circle where you would like to stop, stand up into Wuji Posture, take eight breaths, and your practice is finished.

SUPPLEMENTAL EXERCISE

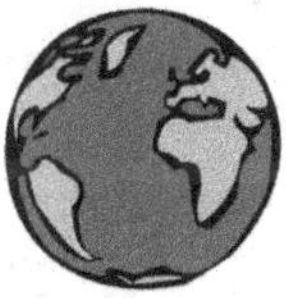

Walking heel-to-toe seems natural enough, but that old enemy, sitting too much, can really interfere with your ability to put one foot in front of the other. What usually happens, is that one foot kicks out sidewise and lands slightly on one side of the foot or the other. You will recognize this when you notice that one shoe is worn excessively on one side. There are many exercise programs that will improve your gait, and I encourage you to explore those.

In the meantime, here are some exercises that I have adapted from traditional Qigong sequences. They focus on the feet section of the Trinity Posture and are designed to remind you that power is generated from the ground up.

FOOT CIRCLES

Foot circles are a staple of many exercise programs. I do mine lying on the floor.

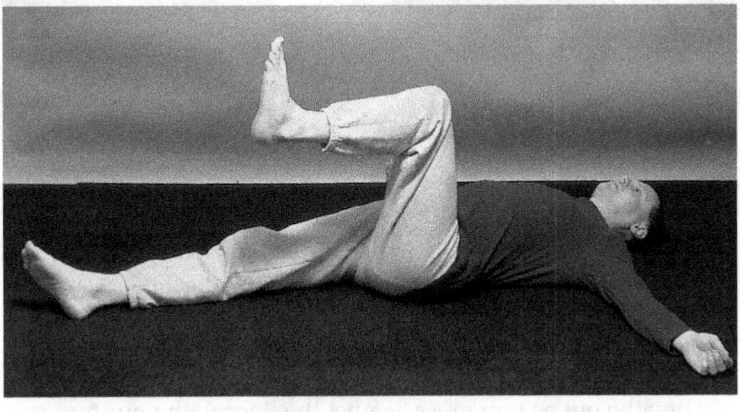

Foot Circles

Lie down on your back with your feet hip width apart and your toes pointing to the ceiling. Stretch your arms out to the sides. Raise the left leg up and bend it at the knee. The position is similar to the Bear Posture, with one leg is raised.

Turn the left foot in circles, first counterclockwise, and then clockwise. Do 30 repetitions in each direction.

When you have finished with the left foot, put the left leg back down, and raise the right leg into the same position. Do 30 Foot Circles in each direction with the right foot before stopping.

THE TURTLE

Lie flat on your stomach (Wuji Posture alignments) with your arms comfortably over your head. Turn your head to the left, so the right cheek and ear are against the floor.

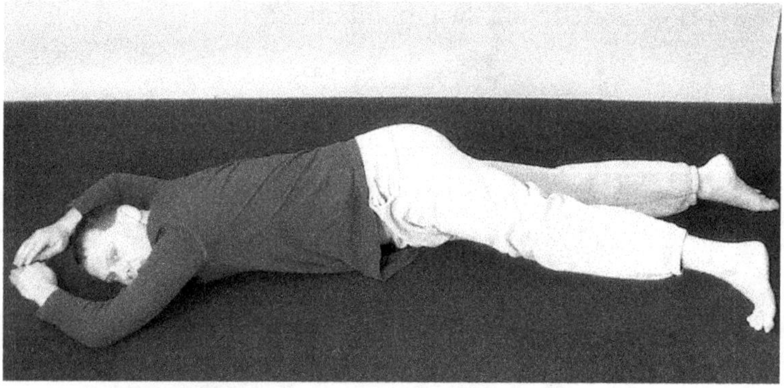

The Turtle

Lift the left foot onto its toes by bending at the ankle. Continue bending at the ankle so you can press against the floor with all the toes of the left foot. Breathe in deeply before continuing.

Breathe out as you press against the floor with your toes and bend the ankle of the left foot as if you were going to take a natural step. The left knee and hip will rise off the floor as you push. Some of the toes of the left foot may come off the floor as well. That is fine, but try to complete the push with all the toes in contact with the floor.

Breathe in as you relax from the push and allow the ankle and toes to settle back into the starting posture. The left knee and hip should fall back on the floor.

Try to keep the right side relaxed as you repeat the entire movement ten times.

When you finish with the left side, repeat the movement on the right side. Remember to turn your head to the right before you curl the toes under and push off of the floor.

This exercise is similar to traditional toe lifts done in a standing posture, but you are focusing on one leg. The lift of the hip and knee that occurs during the push, reminds you that the foot is connected to the torso through the knee and hip.

If this exercise is too strenuous, then traditional toe lifts are fine.

BACK KICK

Lie on your stomach as you did in The Turtle exercise. Turn you face to the left by putting your right cheek and ear against the floor.

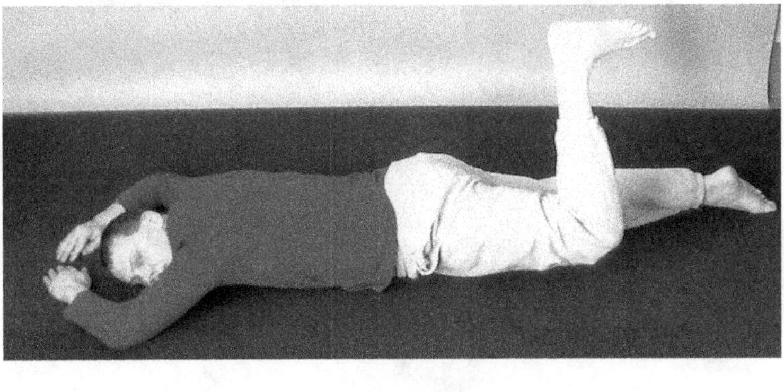

Back Kick

Bend the knee of the left leg so the bottom of the left foot is facing to the ceiling. Take a deep breath, and then breathe out as you push the left foot towards the ceiling by lifting the left thigh off the floor. Hold this position for one minute, before slowly lowering the thigh back to the floor. The right side should remain relaxed while the left side is trying to hold the foot in the air. When your thigh is flat against floor, straighten the leg and recover for a few breaths before you perform the exercise on the other side.

This exercise stresses the link between the foot section and the head section of the Trinity Posture. It reminds you that the performance of your torso, and your legs are linked, and that power flows through the legs and into the torso before it is expressed in the hands.

TRADITIONAL WALKING METHODS

Once you are comfortable walking around the circle with the Natural Step described in the previous section, you can practice two alternate stepping patterns that come from traditional Baguazhang practice.

The first of these is the Sliding Step, and it is probably the most common type of stepping used in Baguazhang. Most schools call this step *walking in mud.* Since it calls for you to walk very slowly, it is good for developing balance and leg strength.

The other method is the Pole Step, and it is also known as a *mud walking* step. It calls for you to lift the entire foot off the floor as one unit and put it down as one unit.

Notice that both stepping patterns are called a *mud walking* step. You could use either version to walk through mud. You could slide your foot along the bottom of a muddy creek, or you could lift the entire foot straight up and out of the mud, while balancing on the other leg. If the goal is to not lose your shoe in the mud, both would probably work, but you might get mud inside your shoe in the process.

Another view of these stepping patterns comes from Chapter 15 of the *Dao De Jing*. Chapter 15 of the *Dao De Jing* describes a true master of Dao. One verse says: "They were careful as someone crossing an iced-over stream." How you choose to cross an iced-over stream depends on the circumstance. If the ice is thick, you may choose to walk over the stream by simply crossing on the ice. However, you will want to test the ice as you step, sliding your foot out, and slowly putting your weight on it. If the ice begins to crack, then you will want to test a different area of the stream before you cross.

If there are rocks in the stream, then you will find that it is safer to cross over by stepping on the rocks. The rocks are small, you can only put one foot on a rock at a time, and the rocks have ice on them as well. You have to put your whole foot down on the rock, and remain balanced on one leg as you walk.

SLIDING STEP

Start in Wuji Posture as before, but instead of putting your left foot down on its heel, lift it slightly, and slide it forward along the floor. The sliding step is not ice skating. You have to lift your foot slightly to slide it along the floor.

Grab the floor with your toes, as you put your weight onto the left foot. Imagine that you are listening for the ice to crack beneath your foot. Do not lift the heel of the right foot.

When all the weight is on the left foot, lift the right foot off the floor slightly and slide it in a path along the edge of the circle. When you have stepped forward with the right foot, begin to put your weight onto it slowly, as you grab the floor with your toes.

Breathe out slowly as you put your weight onto a foot, and breathe in slowly as you move the rear foot next to, and past, the front foot. This means that each foot will take one complete breath (in and out).

POLE STEP

Start in Wuji posture, and put the left foot forward with the sole of the foot flat on the floor. Put your weight onto the left foot and lift the entire right foot off the floor. Bring it next to the left foot and pause for one moment. Then swing the right foot forward and drop the entire foot onto the floor. The pole step is not hopping; it is walking by raising and lowering the entire foot.

Lifting the entire foot off the floor is harder than it sounds. It helps to imagine that your big toe is lifting up first, as if you are kicking something with your toes.

Breathing is similar to the Natural Step; breathe in as you move the inside foot, and breath out as you move the outside foot.

RECOMMENDED PRACTICE

I recommend that you practice all three of these walking patterns, Natural Step, Sliding Step, and Pole Step. Choose one pattern each day and practice it exclusively for that day. Beginners will want to change patterns every day, until all three become natural. When walking the circle is easy for you, then use the Natural Step for most of your practice, and use the Sliding Step and Pole Step once a week.

Once you have committed to a pattern, stick with it, even when you are changing directions. You will find that it is easy to slip into the Natural Step when changing directions, especially if you are practicing the Sliding Step.

STANDING PALMS

Now that you have learned to walk, you will hold increasingly demanding postures with your upper body while walking around the circle. In traditional Baguazhang practice these are called the Basic Palms, or the Standing Palms. The name *Standing Palms* implies that the palms are *standing,* or *fixed* in place while the legs are moving.

Do not underestimate this activity's physical requirement. Circle walking with the fixed upper body postures is a serious exercise program. These postures will stretch and strengthen your torso, challenge your balance, and invigorate you.

I present these Standing Palms in a sequence that calls for an increasing amount of twist in your upper torso. If you cannot perform a posture, you can practice the postures that preceded it until your torso loosens.

Each of the Standing Palms builds on the previous posture, and once you have learned all eight of the Standing Palms you can link the postures by changing from Lowering Palm to Pushing Palm, and so on, as you walk around the circle.

The sequence of eight Standing Palms that I present is my own. Different schools of Baguazhang use different postures for the Standing Palms. Some schools have eight Standing Palms; others may use only one.

The postures and the sequence are less important than the practice. Each of these Standing Palms contributes in some way to the more complex changes that follow. Once you have learned all eight of them, they should be a part of your daily practice.

The number of circles you walk in each posture is your decision, but it should be an equal number in each direction.

LOWERING PALM

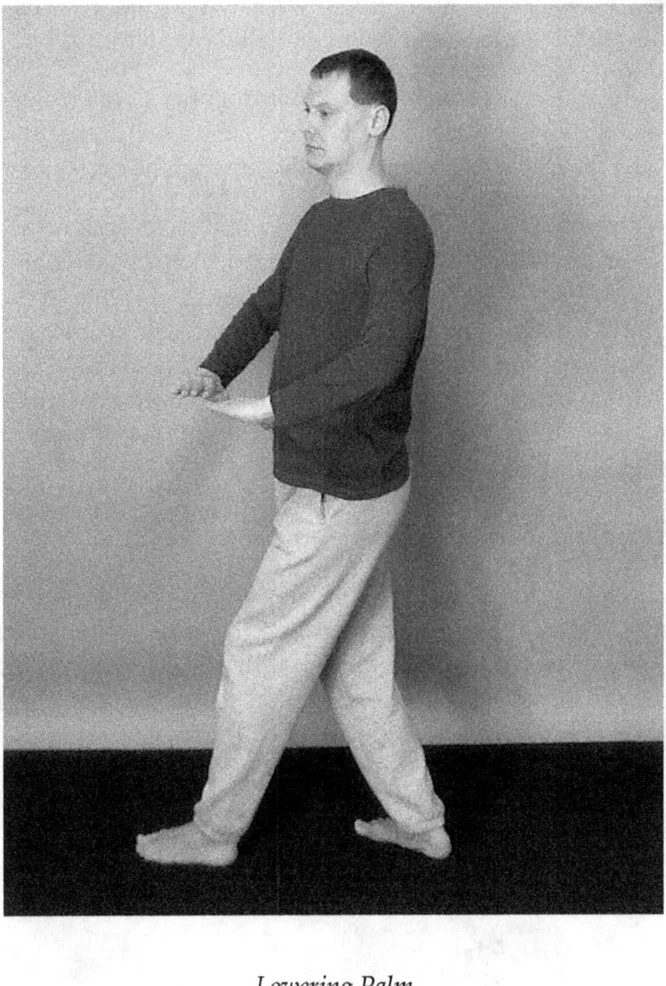

Lowering Palm

Start in Wuji Posture facing in the counterclockwise direction on your circle. Raise your hands to the height of your belly button with the palms facing down. Remember the lessons from Holding the Moon Posture in your standing exercise. The shoulders and elbows need to have that sinking feeling, without rolling forward and down. There will be a gap between your outstretched fingers that should correspond to the center line of your body. Turn to the center of the circle with your torso, but keep your hands in front of you. You can imagine that you are holding a ball under water with your palms as you walk.

When you have walked a certain number of circles in the counterclockwise direction, perform a Simple Change while keeping the upper torso turned to the center of the circle.

Being able to hold the upper body in a fixed position while your feet maneuver under you is a great advantage, and one that we engage in without thinking. Consider carrying a large object--like a television set--up a flight of stairs, down a long narrow hallway, and into your apartment, or bedroom. You will have to twist and turn your torso and feet at different times to maneuver the television through narrow doorways, over stair railings, and onto a counter top.

PUSHING PALM

This posture is the Holding the Moon Posture, but your palms are facing outward. By twisting the arms you are engaging the muscles along their entire length and encouraging interactions with supporting muscles in the torso. You can imagine that a large ball is pushing against you, and you are resisting with your palms.

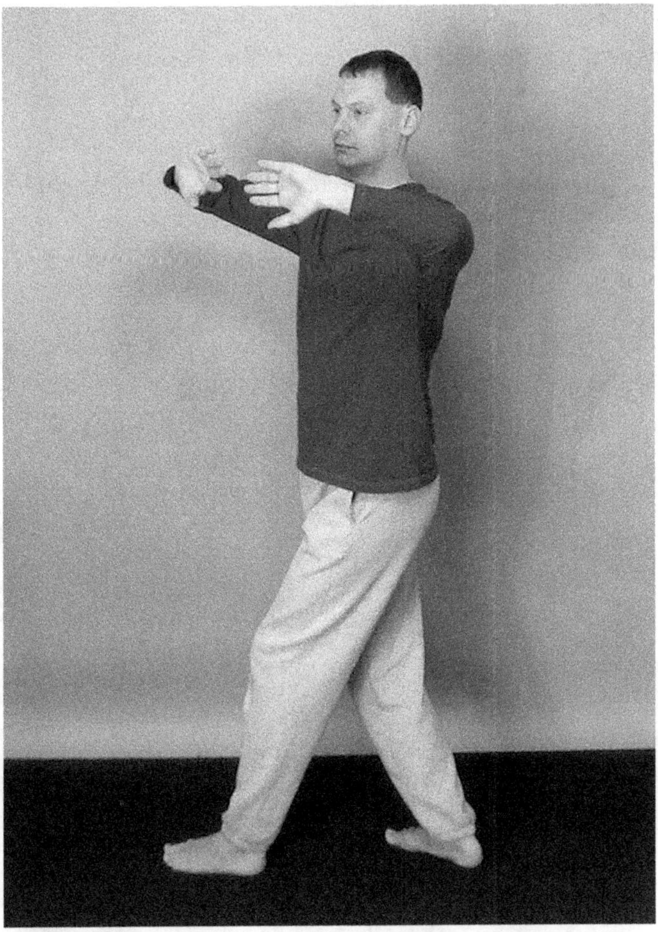

Pushing Palm

Stand on the edge of the circle in the Wuji Posture. Start in the Lowering Palm Posture, then raise your palms to shoulder height.

This posture can cause your shoulders and head to rise. Try to relax and remember the alignments of Wuji Posture. Your shoulders should remain back, not rounded forward, and the crown of your head should feel as if it is being pulled up by a string, causing your chin to tuck in and down.

Walk as before, and change direction with the Simple Change while maintaining the upper body posture.

HOLDING THE FRUIT PALM

Begin on the edge of the circle in Pushing Palm posture, then turn the palms upward by sinking the elbows down. It is important to make this movement from the elbows. If you make it from the shoulders, you will roll your shoulders forward.

As you lower your elbows and turn your palms upward bring the hands together so they are touching below the pinkies;

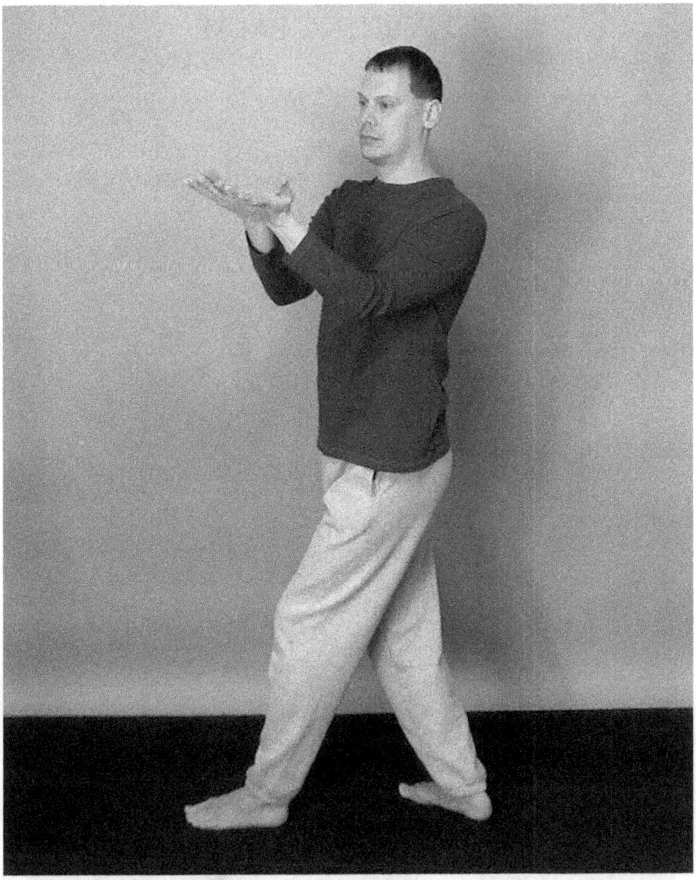

Holding the Fruit Palm

the pinkies are not touching each other. Do not smash the hands with force; they should touch gently or be just a hair's breadth apart.

Walk and change direction as before.

SUPPORTING PALM

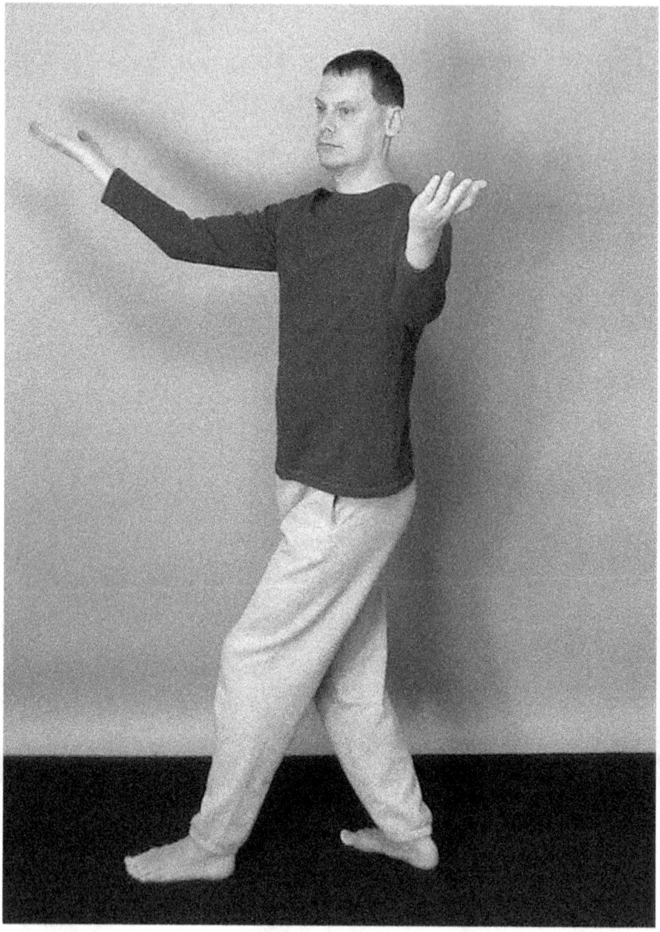

Supporting Palm

The Supporting Palm is a classic posture in Baguazhang practice. In some schools, the only fixed posture practice is Supporting Palm.

Start from Holding The Fruit Palm and then push your palms from you in the direction of your thumbs. This will be slightly more than 45 degrees, but less than 90 degrees from the plane of your shoulders.

Keep your palms upright. You may find that it is harder to keep one palm facing up than the other, or that one palm turns over slightly when you change direction. Imagine that you are holding a ball or a cup of hot tea in each hand as you walk the circle.

Walk and change direction as before.

ROLLING THE BALL PALM

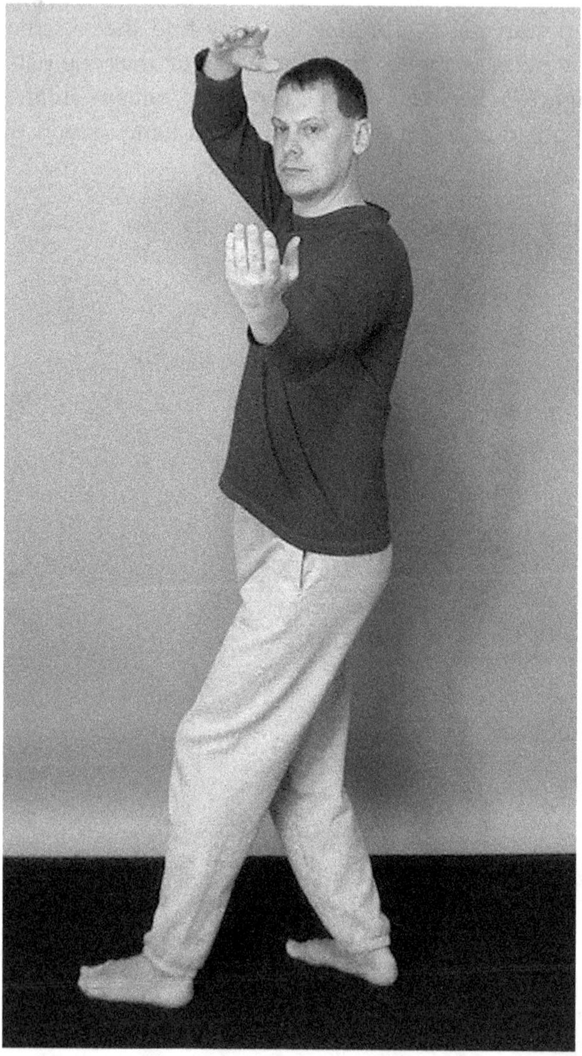

Rolling the Ball Palm

Rolling the Ball Palm is an excellent exercise for your torso. It is also the first posture that requires you to change hand positions as you perform the Simple Change. Stand on the edge of the circle facing in the counterclockwise direction. Assume the Supporting Palm posture and then lift the right arm up and over the head so the right palm is facing down, and the fingers are pointing to the center of the circle. The image is that you are holding a large ball into the center of the circle as you walk around it.

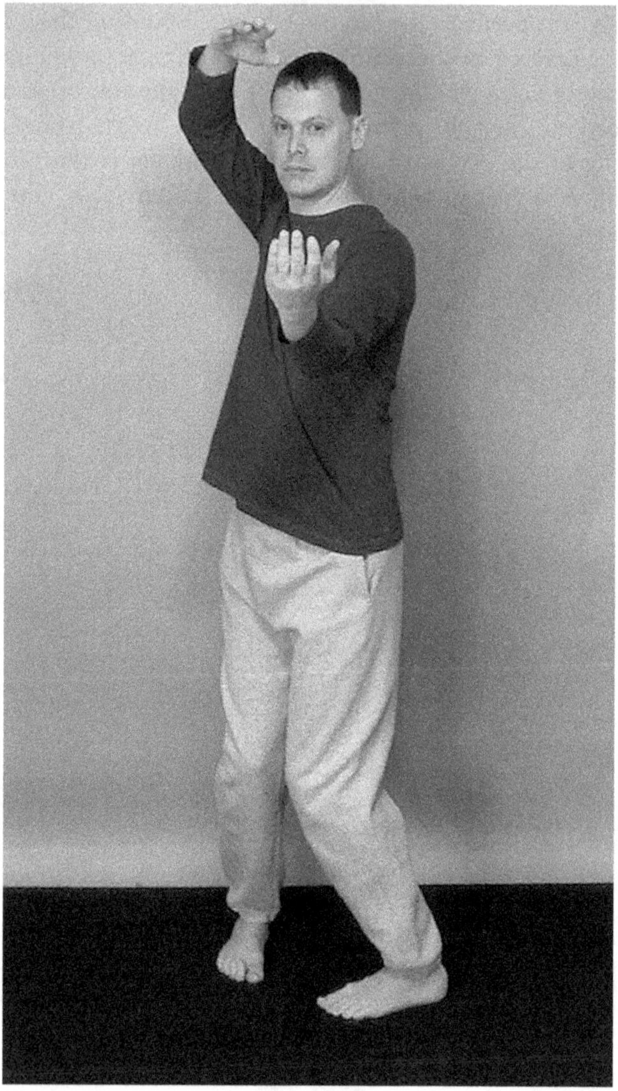

Rolling the Ball Palm -- toe-in

Walk as before, but when you toe-in for the Simple Change

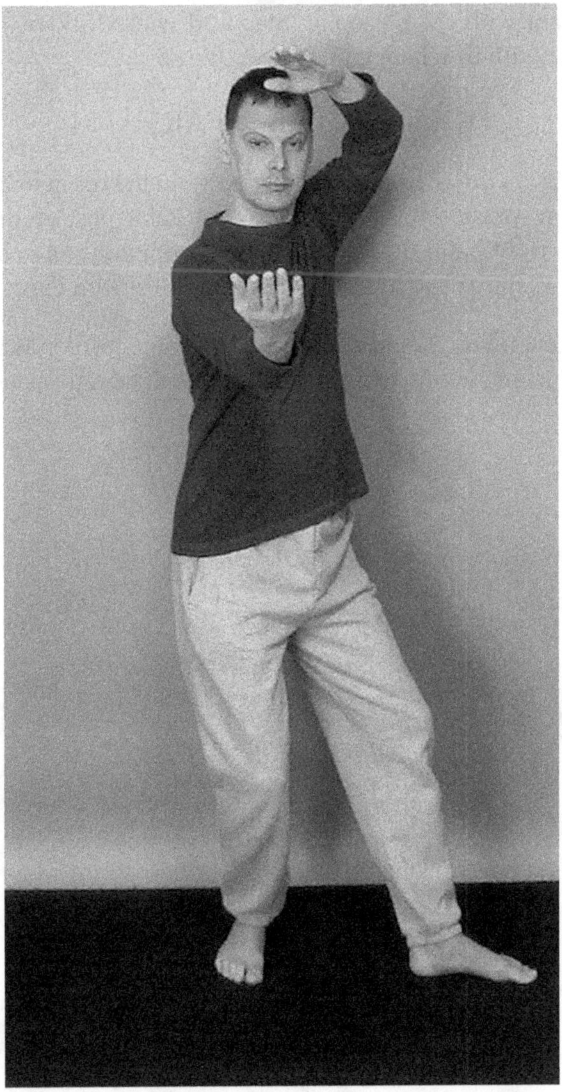

Rolling the Ball Palm -- toe-out

maintain the posture, with the left hand pointing directly to the center of the circle. Then roll your hands along the edge of your imaginary ball as you toe-out. Complete the Simple Change movement with the Sweeping Step and walk clockwise around the circle with the changed posture.

HOLDING THE SPEAR PALM

Stand on the edge of the circle facing in the counterclockwise direction. Assume the Rolling the Ball Palm posture and then turn the right palm over so it is facing from you. As you turn it over, bend the elbow so the right palm is level with the forehead.

Another way to find the right hand palm position is to stand in the Pushing Palm posture and then raise the right hand to the

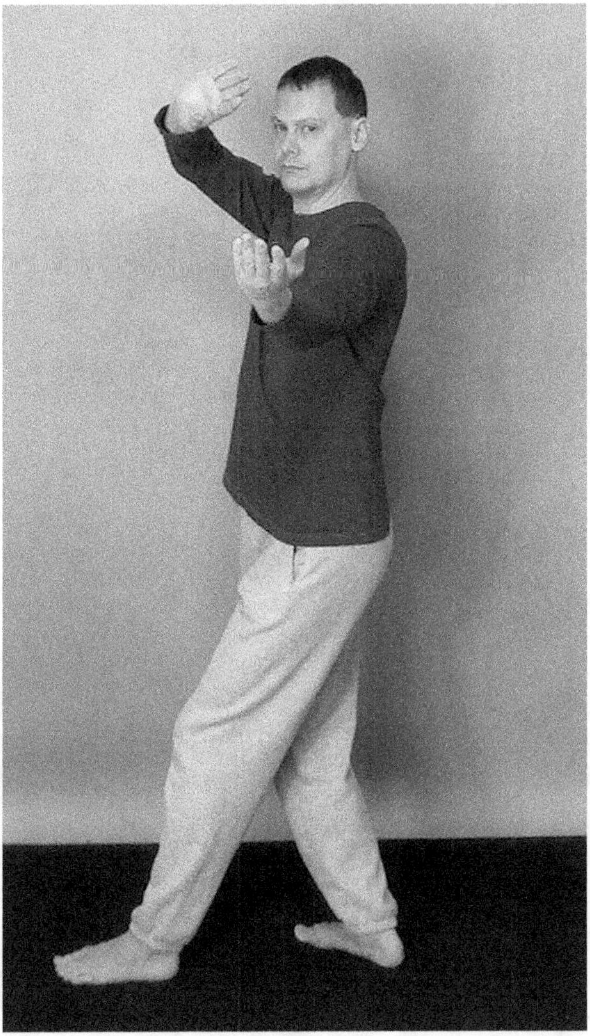

Holding the Spear Palm

forehead. The left hand remains in its Supporting Palm position. The image is that you are holding a spear between the thumb and forefinger of both hands.

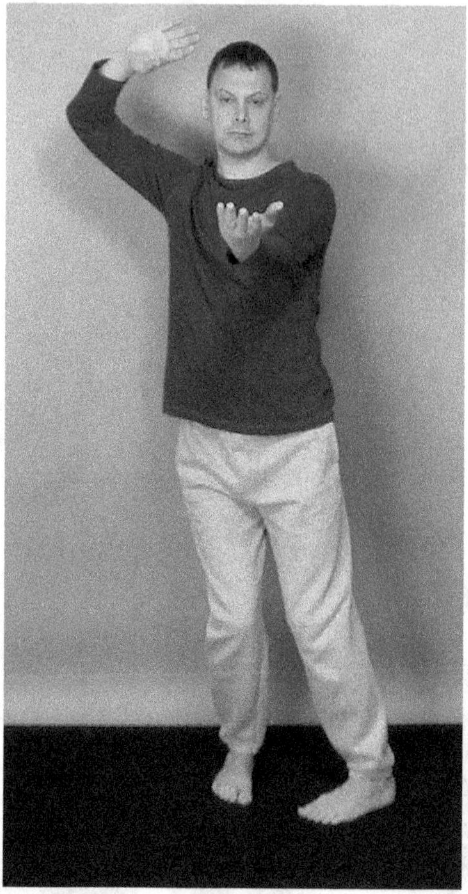

Holding the Spear Palm -- toe-in

Perform the Simple Change as before, but maintain the

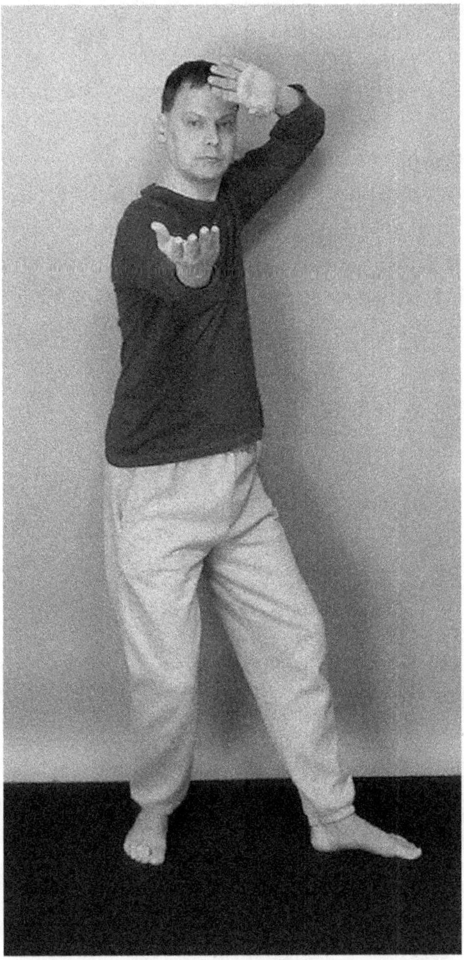

Holding the Spear Palm -- toe-out

palm positions when you toe-in. The right hand will appear to move from the forehead as your torso turns. When you toe-out, move both hands in an arc so that the left hand replaces the right at the forehead, and the right extends to the center of the circle.

SKY AND GROUND PALM

Stand on the edge of the circle facing in the counterclockwise direction. From Holding the Spear Posture lower the right hand down the front of the body with the palm facing away, while the left hand rises from its extended position with the palm facing to the body. You can over stretch this posture by raising the left shoulder and straightening the left elbow. If you want to maintain the Wuji Posture alignments, you will not straighten the left elbow. I prefer the latter posture, but either is acceptable.

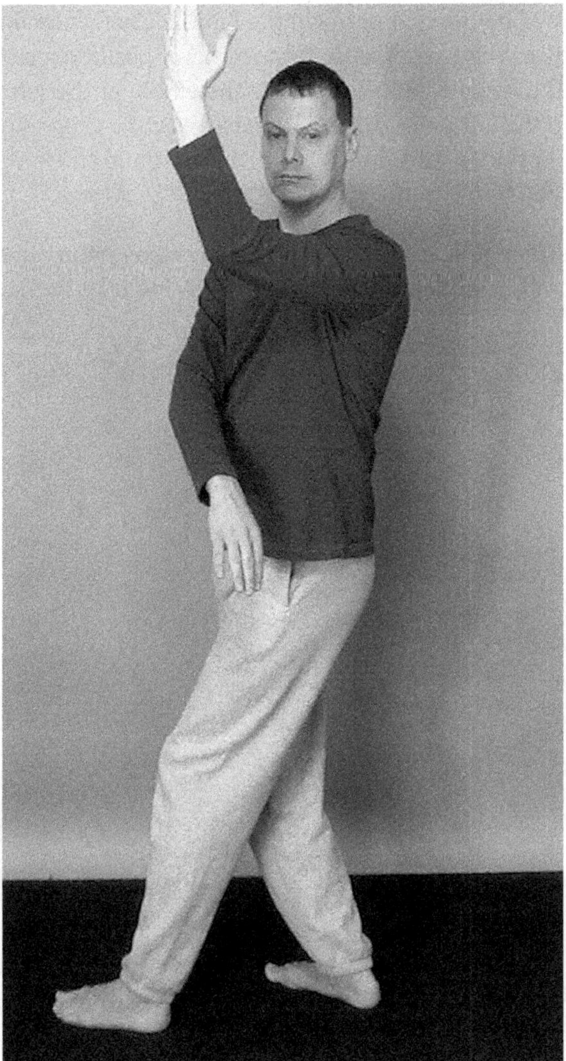

Sky and Ground Palm

Walk as before and perform the Simple Change, maintaining the posture when you toe-in. Change hand positions as you toe-out. Drill the right palm up, inside the elbow of the left arm, as you drop the left palm down. As the arms change positions they twist in opposite directions. The arms continue to change positions as you perform the Sweeping Step.

This change is different from the previous palms in that the arms do not complete their change until you take the Sweeping Step.

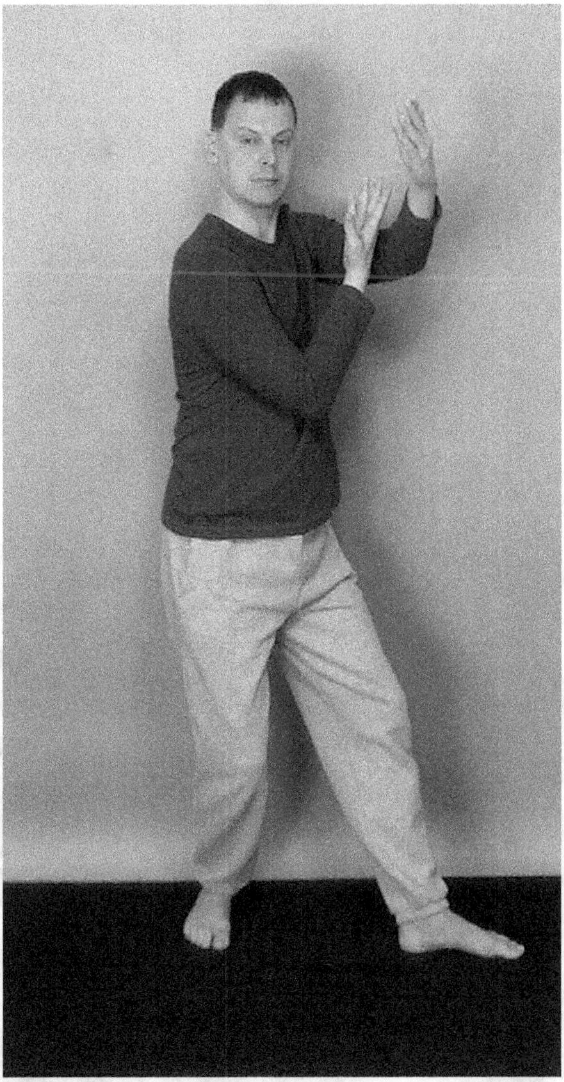

Sky and Ground Palm -- toe-out

PUSHING MILLSTONE PALM

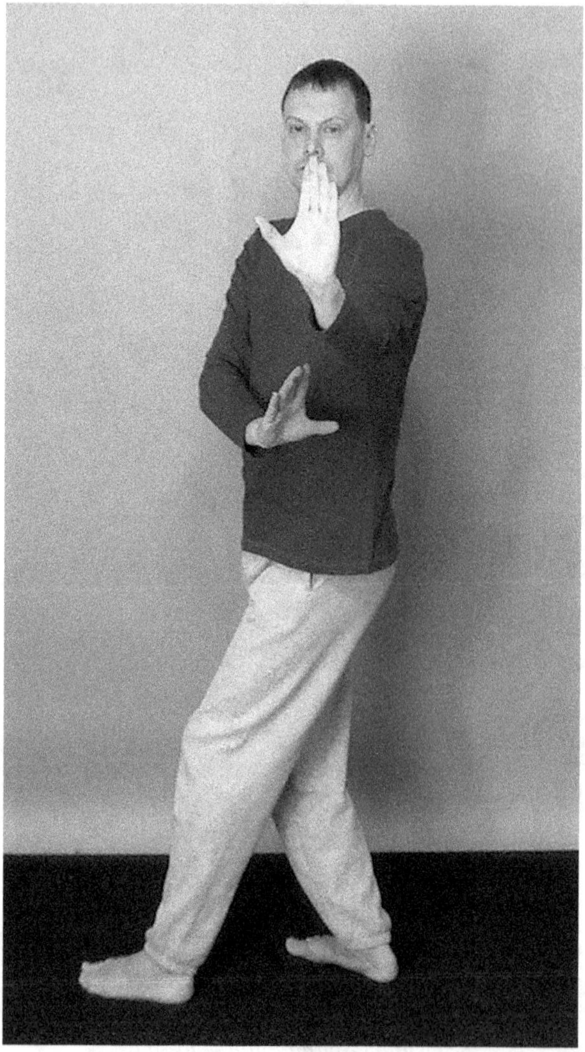

Pushing Millstone Palm

The last Standing Palm posture is the main posture for Baguazhang practice, and you can add it as a fifth posture for your standing practice.

Assume the left Yin Yang Posture on the edge of the circle facing in the counterclockwise direction. Drop the heel of the left foot and place your hands into the Trinity Posture positions. Then turn your upper body so the forefinger of the left hand aligns with the center of the circle.

The right hand will move naturally to the left as you turn. Bend the elbow of the right arm, and stand the right hand up so that the fingers are under the left elbow. It is easy to pull the right shoulder forward when assuming this posture; do not. Keep the shoulders in the Wuji Posture alignment.

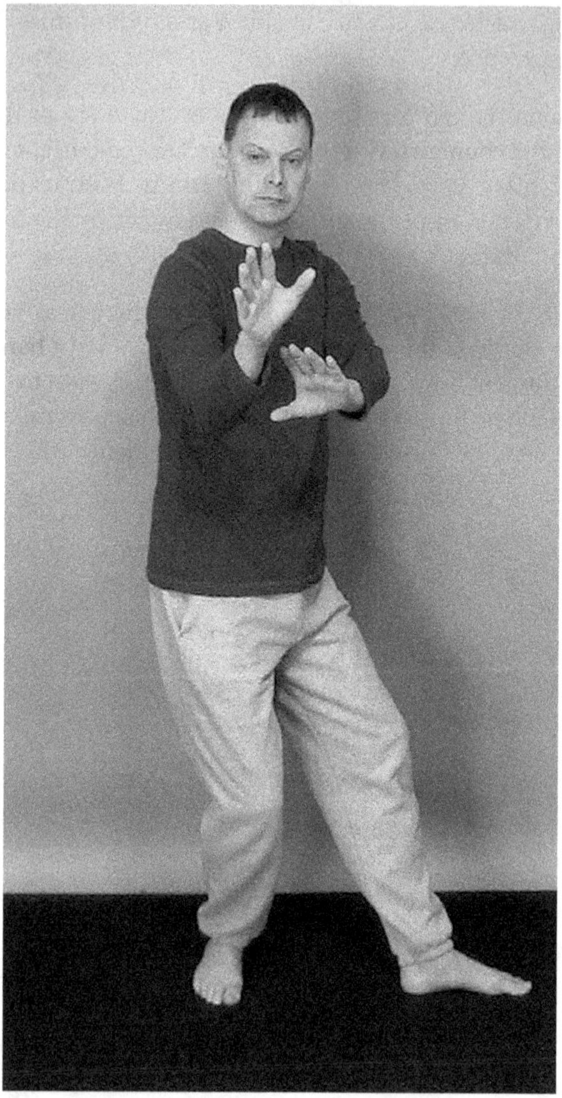

Pushing Millstone Palm -- toe-out

Walk the circle and perform a Simple Change. The right hand pierces under the left hand, and the left hand pulls back to the waist as you toe-out. Imagine that you are tearing a piece of cloth as you make this change.

SUPPLEMENTAL EXERCISE

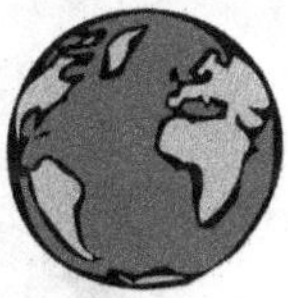

Turning at the torso is not something we do everyday. As you progress through these postures, you will notice a difference in your overall agility as your torso loosens, and you gain balance. Here are two exercises that will loosen and strengthen the torso and speed your progress.

FLOOR TWIST

The Floor Twist is one of my favorite exercises. It has made a significant difference in my Baguazhang practice.

Lie on your left side with the left arm stretched straight out to the left and the palm facing up. Stretch your right arm out along your left with the palm down. Pull your knees up and straighten the lower legs. This posture is similar to the Bear Posture, but on your side.

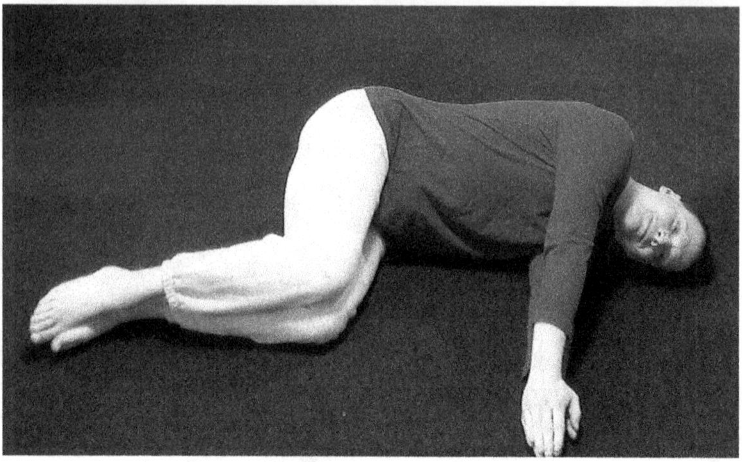

Floor Twist -- One

Turn to your right moving the right arm in a large arc over your head so it comes to rest on the floor with the palm facing up. Let your upper torso and head follow the movement of the hand. Prevent your knees from sliding or rising up by using your left hand to catch and hold them in place.

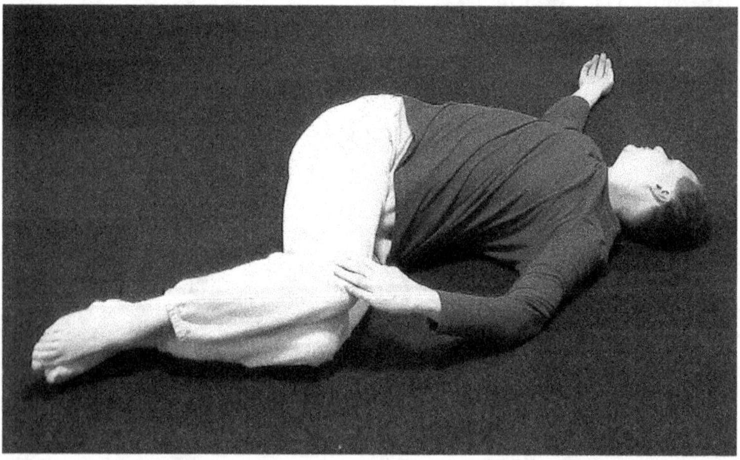

Floor Twist -- Two

This can be a significant stretch for most people, so go slowly. You may want to start by sliding the right hand along the left arm as you turn your torso; turn your torso and head until the right elbow touches the floor.

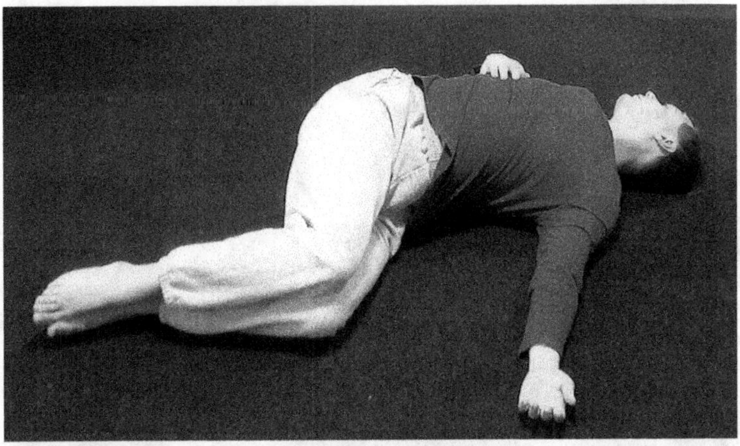

Floor Twist -- Partial

Hold the position for one minute before bringing the right arm back to its starting position, then roll over and repeat the entire exercise on your right side.

CRUNCHES

The Standing Palm practice is a traditional method to build strength and flexibility in the torso. Here is another traditional exercise for your torso, and one of the most hated words in the English language, Crunches.

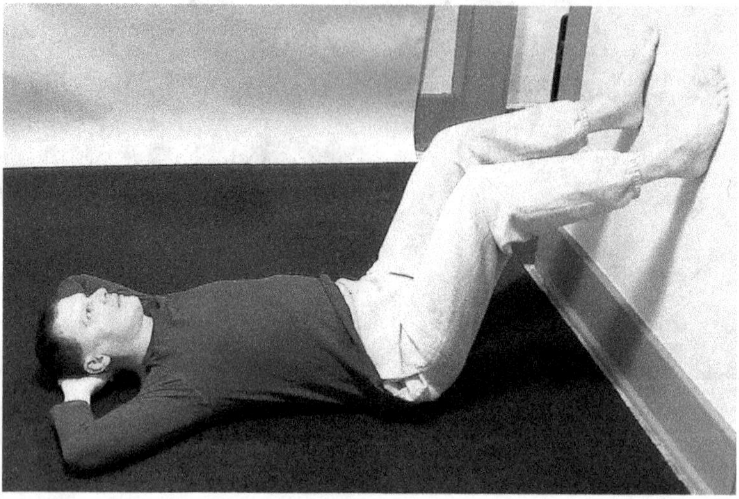

Crunches -- One

Lie in the Bear Posture with your feet against a wall. Put your hands under your head and take a deep breath.

Breathe out as you lift your shoulders and head off the floor. Keep your eyes focused on the ceiling; if you can see the wall your feet are against, then you have lifted too far off the floor. Hold the position for just one moment, then breathe in as you lie back down.

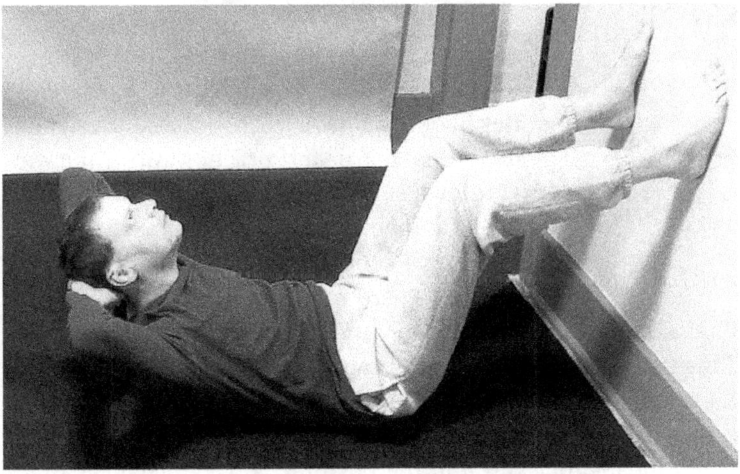

Crunches -- Two

As you lift up, be sure that your elbows do not curl forward around your ears; keep them pulled back. Also, do not leverage your Crunch with your feet; all the work should be done by the muscles in the lower torso.

One set is 25 repetitions.

EIGHT TRIGRAM PALM

If you have been practicing the exercises in this book, you have learned the fundamentals to internal martial art practice. Along the way, you have supplemented the traditional training with the floor exercises that reinforced the traditional concepts. With this information in hand, you are ready to practice the classical Baguazhang forms described in Sun Lu Tang's book. Sun Lu Tang named this Baguazhang practice method as *Swimming Body Eight Trigrams Connected Palms. Swimming Body* implies that the postures are performed in a continuous manner, while *Connected Palms* means that you link the postures with the changes in direction. Do not think of the forms in this section as a routine that you must practice one after another, rather as characters of an alphabet that you can connect to create your own routines.

Before you can achieve the free form practice of *Swimming Body Connected Palms,* however, you must work on the basics of learning the postures. First, you should practice slowly, performing each change of direction with care. Pause at each step to check your body alignment, much as you did in Standing and Standing Palms practice. When you feel comfortable with your body alignments, you can move through the changes with slight pauses at the extremes of each posture. Sun Lu Tang reinforced this image in his book by saying that the "posture stops, but it does not stop." Think of water moving inside a bag as you shake it. When you stop shaking the bag, the water continues to move about, causing the bag to move. After much practice you will be able to change directions without thinking and move from one change to another in a continuous manner.

Once you have attained the highest level of practice, you cannot abandon the basics. At the end of this book is a Recommended Practice section that provides some hints on staying in touch with the basics as you progress in skill.

MARTIAL APPLICATIONS

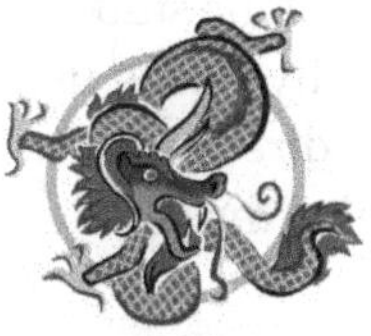

I talked a little bit about meditation in the Attention section of the this book. By practicing Attention with the physical exercises of this book, you have a tool to achieve a higher state of mind than most people around you. The biggest side effect of this attention is that you will be more aware of the present moment--your surroundings, and the current situation--than those around you. You will notice people with bad posture, or people who are not breathing. You will recognize situations that seem like a major crises to others as imagined obstacles that do not exist in the now.

This attention to the present moment is the single most important teaching of any pugilistic skill. Without presence, you cannot win a fight. Someone that is not present in a fight will be thinking about all the past harms their opponent has done them, and use those memories to fuel their rage. Others may be focused on how cool they will be after they have kicked their opponent's ass, and what a great story their defeat will make.

The trained boxer, on the other hand, defeats himself first. He recognizes that fighting will benefit no one. Someone will get hurt, and there can be no awareness at the moment of doing harm. Attention recognizes that all the perceived hurts or imagined victories do not exist, NOW. The practiced martial artist does not seek to harm, but to return safely from the encounter. Ultimately that is the real struggle of life--return safely from the encounter.

Circle walking is the method used in applying Baguazhang for martial purposes. There is an old saying, "The hands defend; the feet win." Circle walking in Baguazhang practice is the continuous training of footwork skills. The ability to change hand positions and defend or attack while moving is a skill that few have.

Books describing martial arts often show martial applications with the description of the posture. The idea is that understanding the form's purpose in a fight will help in your study of the posture and improve your practice of it. Usually this is useful, since many martial forms have evident and direct applications. Baguazhang, however, is about change, and the applications are less evident.

Martial art instructors have devised many ways to preserve and transmit the martial applications of an art. The most popular method is the practice of Pushing Hands. Pushing Hands is a two-person training routine that teaches leverage, sensitivity, positioning, and coordination. Another method is the use of key words that describe the fighting essence of the art.

Instead of looking for specific applications in the Baguazhang postures, consider these key words and how each of them could be applied at any instant in your circle walking practice.

The Eight Abilities (Key Words) are:

- *Parry:* Ward off the opponent's hand, foot, shoulder or hip with a countermove. Similar to Block, But you do not rub the opponent.

- *Block:* Hinder or stop the opponent's movement or action by rubbing against the hand or foot of the opponent with your hand, shoulder, hip, or foot.

- *Intercept:* Prevent an opponent's strike from landing by deflecting it with a hand, elbow, shoulder, or hip. Parry is round, Intercept is straight.

- *Knock:* Collide with the opponent's breast or abdomen with your elbow, shoulder, hip, or knee.

- *Push:* Use one or both hands to hold or exert force against the opponent. This is also called a strike.

- *Uphold:* Lift the opponent's hands away from the intended strike.

• *Carry:* When grabbed by the opponent, support the grab and move to break the hold. This may be done by Knocking, Upholding, or Lifting.

• *Lift:* Raise or lower the opponent's body, causing their balance to be lost.

PRACTICE METHOD

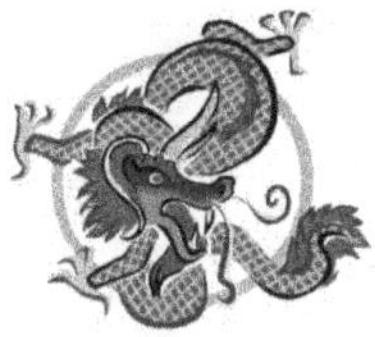

When practicing the postures described in this section, use the Natural Step to walk around the circle. Walk slowly, pausing with each step to check your body alignment. Pictures and descriptions are for the left turning (walking in the counterclockwise direction with the left hand in the center of the circle) changes only. Reverse the descriptions to perform the change on the right side. Perform each change an equal number of times for both the left and right hands.

Sun Lu Tang connected each of the twelve postures in his book to a concept from Daoist cosmology. You are familiar with the first two postures.

Wuji: Before you begin practice, stand in Wuji posture. (*See* Wuji Posture on page 53.)

Taiji: Before you begin to move there is the intention of moving, and then there is the separation of Yin and Yang. Before you begin to walk the circle, stand in the Pushing Millstone posture on the edge of the circle. This announces your intention to move and create Yin and Yang. (*See* Pushing Millstone Palm on page 104.)

SINGLE PALM CHANGE

Liang Yi: Liang Yi is the two poles of Yin and Yang. In Baguazhang walking to the left (counterclockwise) is Yang, walking to the right (clockwise) is Yin. Sun Lu Tang associated the Single Palm Change to Liang Yi.

From the left Pushing Millstone Palm, toe-in with the right foot to begin the change. The torso posture does not change.

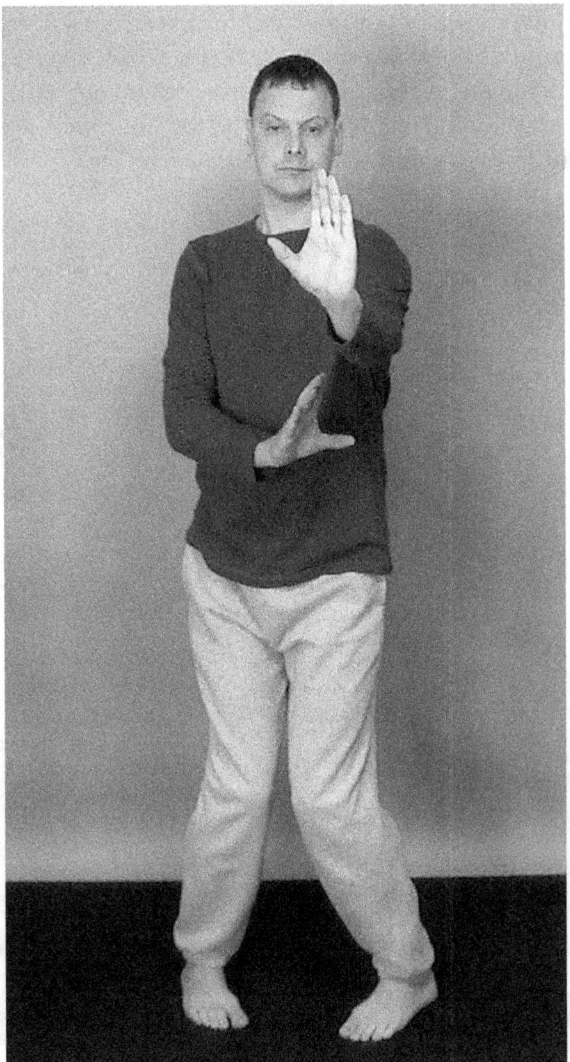

Single Palm Change -- One

Toe-out with the right foot and turn the palms over so they are pushing in the direction of the change. This movement can look as if you are pushing with the arms but do not; maintain the torso and arm alignments and let the toe-out movement create the push. The eyes remain focused on the left hand.

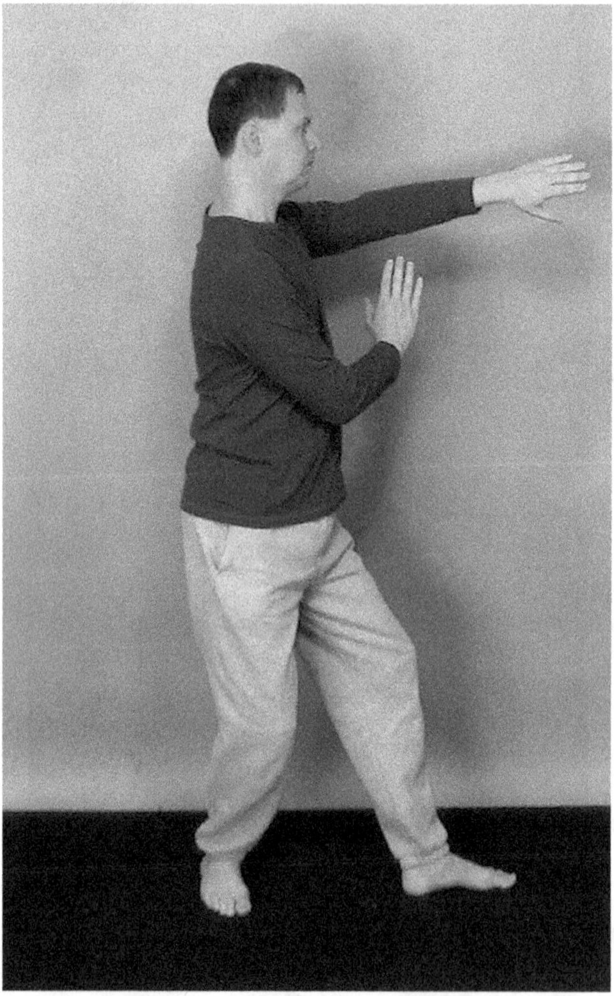

Single Palm Change -- Two

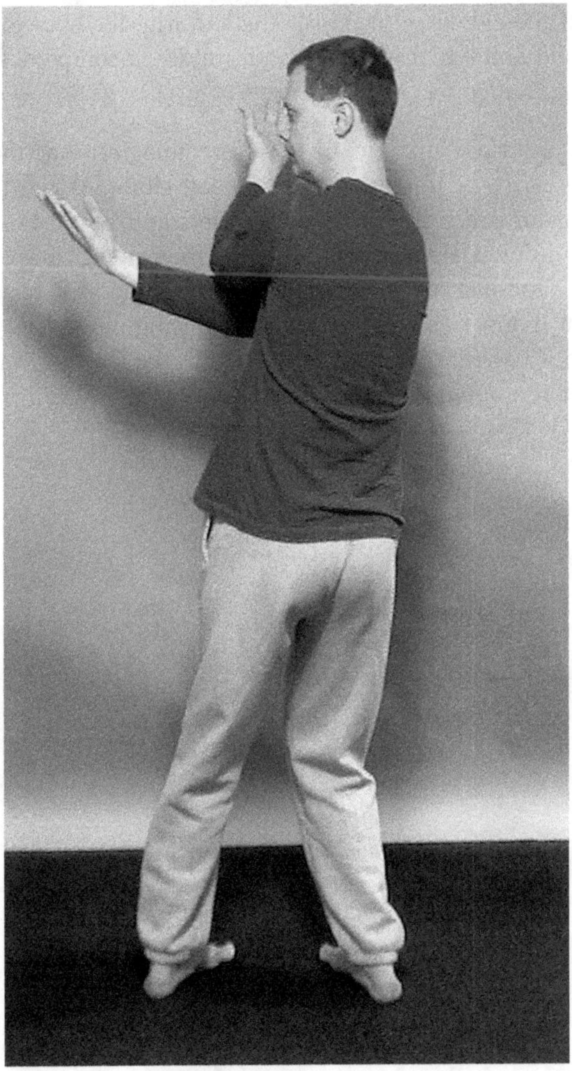

Single Palm Change -- Three

Toe-in with the right foot so the body is facing from the center of the circle. The right hand pierces under the left elbow with the palm facing up. The left palm turns over to face upwards as the right hand pierces under the elbow. The arms form a "T" shape at the elbow. As it passes the left arm, the eyes catch the right hand and remain focused on it until you complete the Single Palm Change.

As you close up into this posture imagine that the right shoulder is trying to pierce under the left elbow. This is the first time in your practice when the shoulders and back can roll forward and down. Remember the rolling movement you practiced with The Bellows, the shoulders and spine should roll forward in a similar manner as you perform this closing movement of Single Palm Change. Your body is twisted to the left like a rope or spring that is about to come undone.

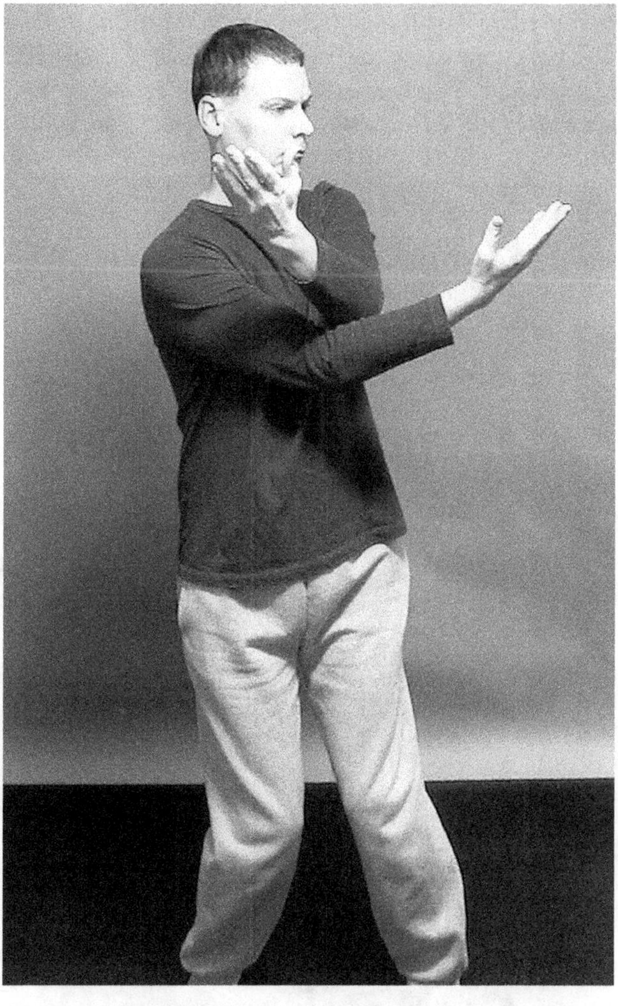

Single Palm Change -- Three (Front)

Let the energy of the coiled rope or spring be released by continuing the pierce of the right hand past the left arm and above the head. The left hand is inside the elbow of the of the right arm, and follows the elbow as you uncoil to the right.

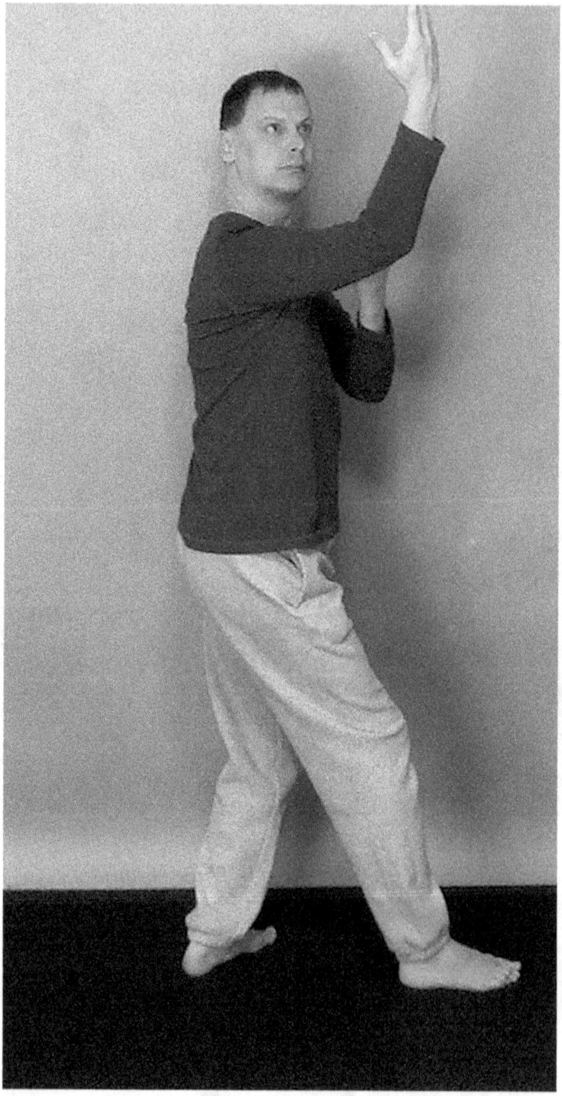

Single Palm Change -- Four

The Single Palm Change completes with a toe-out of the right foot as your right and left hand lower into the Pushing Millstone Posture.

Begin walking in the clockwise direction by Stealing a Step with the right foot and then following with a Sweep Step of the left foot along the line of the circle.

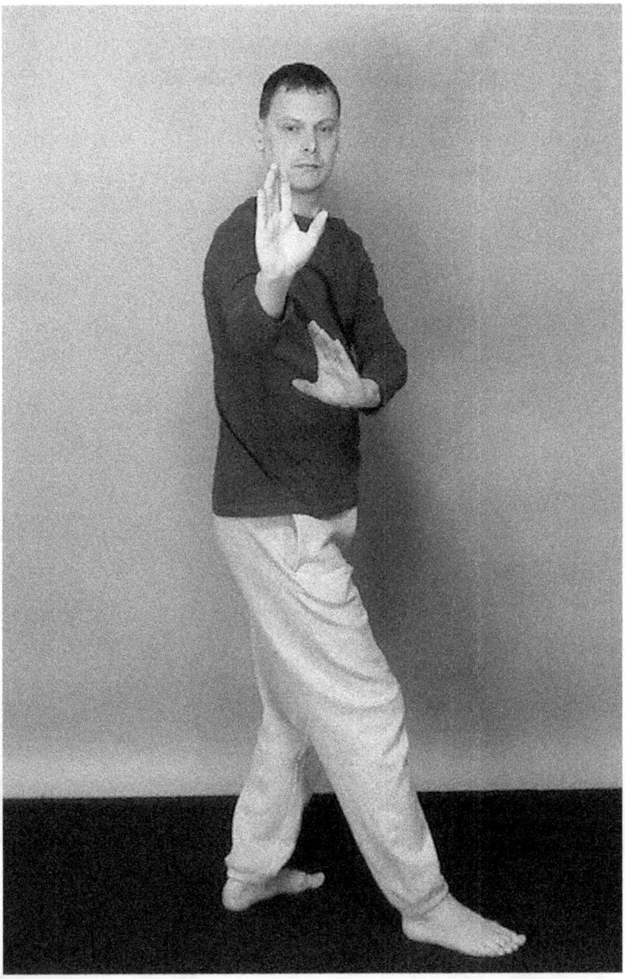

Single Palm Change -- Five

Walk at least three circles before changing directions with a right turning Single Palm Change.

DOUBLE PALM CHANGE

Si Xiang: Si Xiang is the transformation (or doubling) of Yin and Yang into Old Yin, Young Yin, Young Yang, and Old Yang. Sun Lu Tang associated Si Xiang with the Double Palm Change.

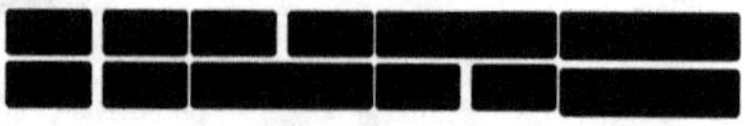

From the left Pushing Millstone Palm toe-in with the right foot to begin the change. The torso posture does not change.

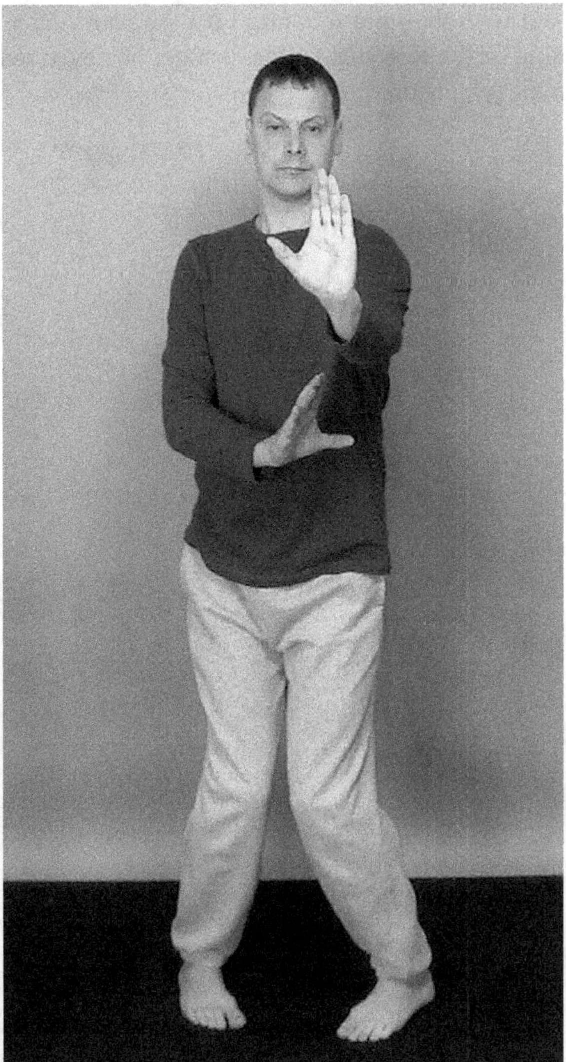

Double Palm Change -- One

Toe-out with the right foot and turn the palms over so they are pushing in the direction of the change. The eyes remain focused on the left hand.

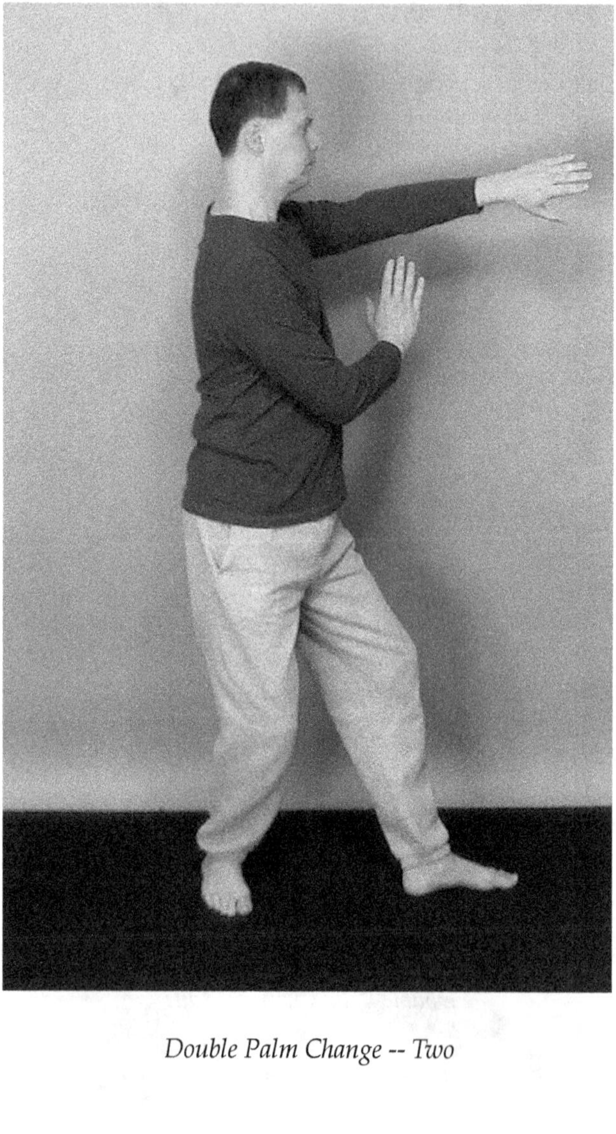

Double Palm Change -- Two

Toe-in with the right foot as you rub the back of the right hand along the inside of the left elbow. Your eyes catch the right hand as it pierces past the elbow.

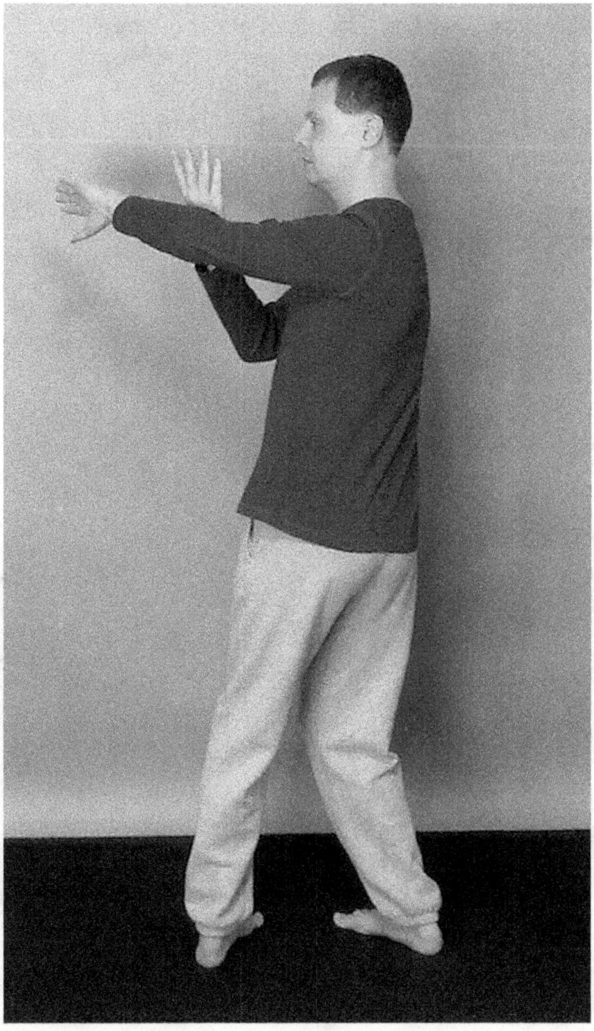

Double Palm Change -- Three

Pierce the right hand above your head as you spin on the ball of the right foot so you are facing in the opposite direction, and slightly to the center of the circle. The left foot comes off the floor as you spin and rests next to the ankle of the right foot. The hands form the Sky and Ground Palm posture in front of the body.

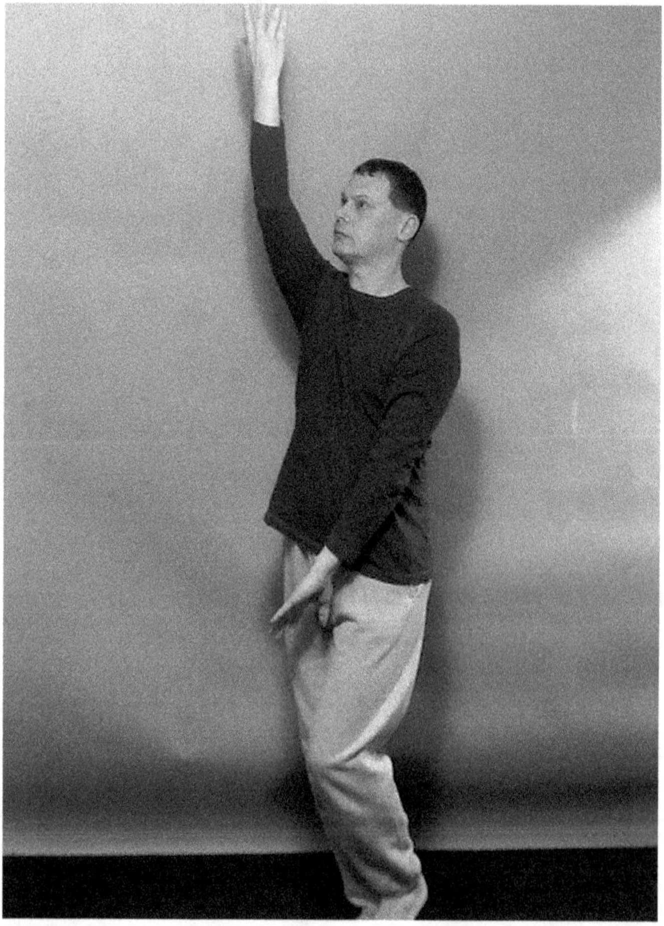

Double Palm Change -- Four

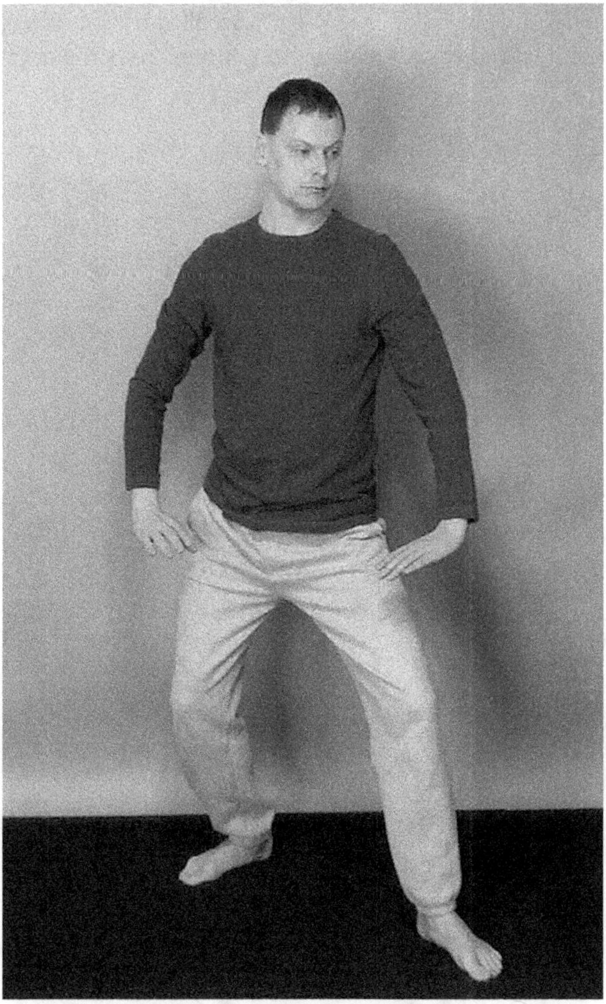

Double Palm Change -- Five

Lower the right hand by swinging it from the shoulder, and raise the left hand by bending the left elbow. The left foot steps out, and your torso is facing the center of the circle; your eyes catch the left hand as your right hand drops past it. The hands, elbows, and knees move in unison as you step out with the left foot. The hands are in the Lowering Palm posture, but held wide, over the thighs of each leg. The elbows, shoulders, and hips are all rounded and feel as though they are sinking into the ground.

Turn the left foot out on its heel, and raise the hands to the pushing position of Single Palm Change.

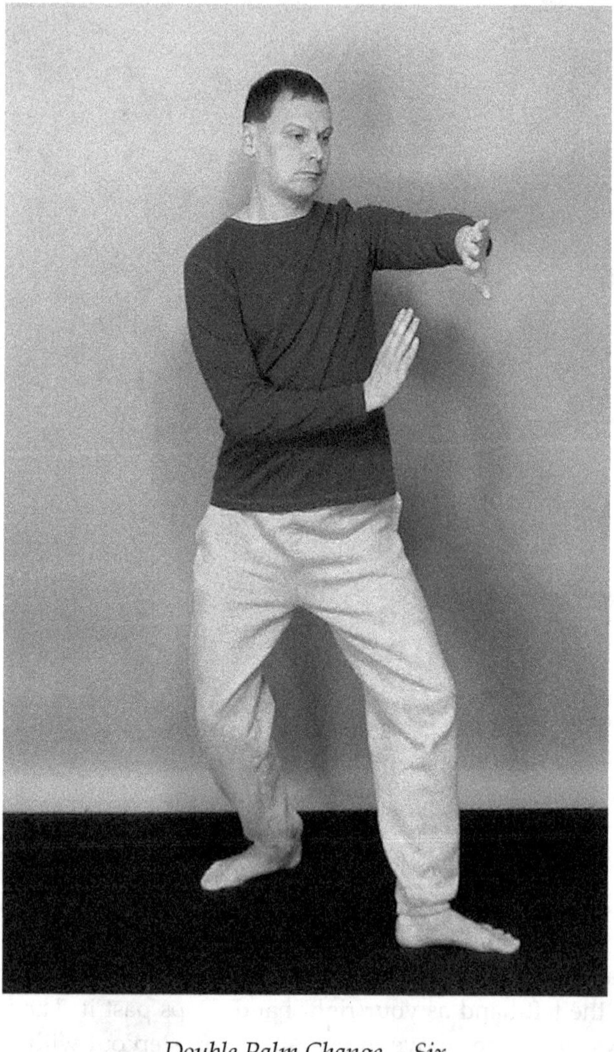

Double Palm Change -- Six

Toe-in with the right foot so the body is facing from the center of the circle. The right hand pierces under the left arm at the elbow. As it passes the left arm, the eyes catch the right hand and remain focused on it until you complete Double Palm Change.

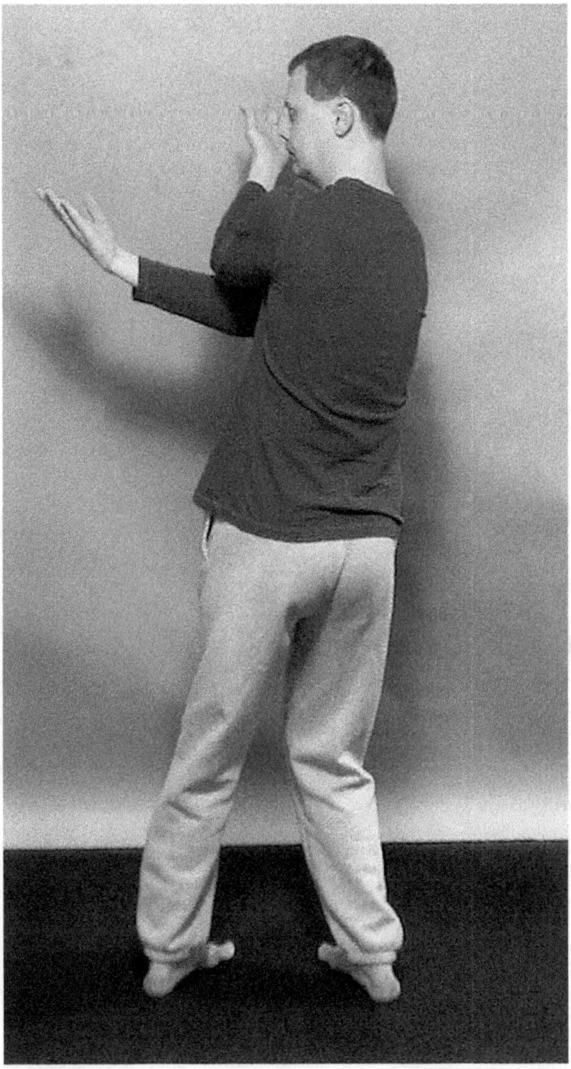

Double Palm Change -- Seven

The right hand continues past the left arm until the right hand is above the head. The left hand is inside the elbow of the of the right arm, and follows the elbow as you uncoil to the right.

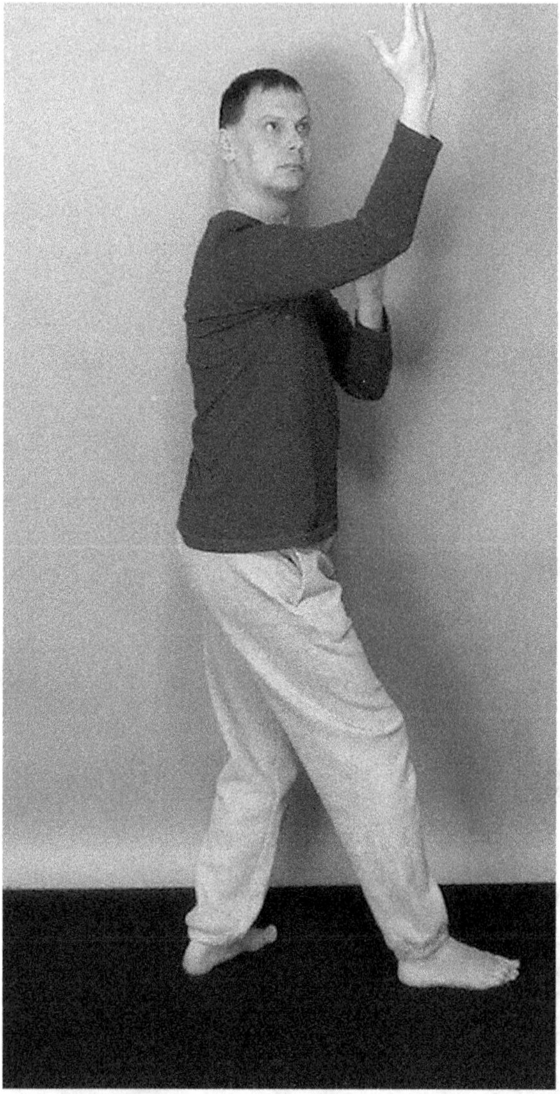

Double Palm Change -- Eight

The Double Palm Change completes with a toe-out of the right foot as your right and left hand lower to the Pushing Millstone Posture.

Begin walking in the clockwise direction by Stealing a Step forward with the right foot and following with a Sweep Step of the left foot along the line of the circle.

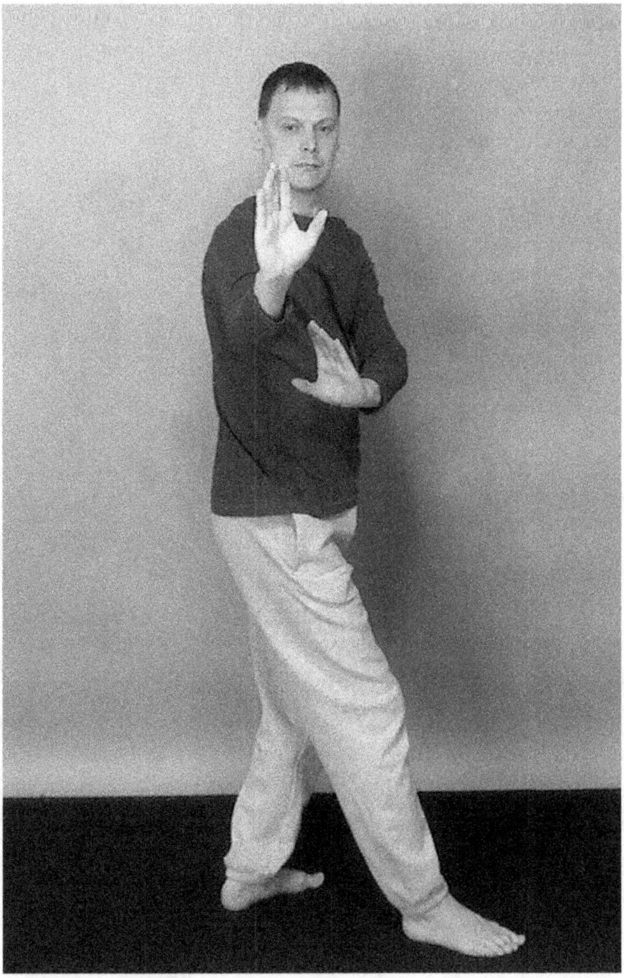

THE TRIGRAMS

Remember the pre-heaven and post-heaven Bagua circles? These two representations of the Bagua trigrams are joined to form the *Pre-Heaven and Post-Heaven Combined As One* representation.

Sun Lu Tang compared good Baguazhang practice to this diagram. You are already familiar with this association, we dis-

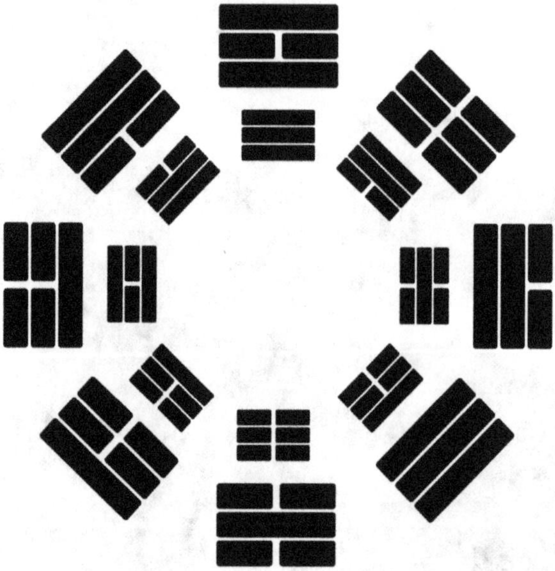

cussed it with the Trinity Posture as the Six Harmonies. Remember that there were three external harmonies (the post-heaven Bagua) and the three internal harmonies (the pre-heaven Bagua). Internal martial art practice requires the study of this relationship between the inner and outer.

LION

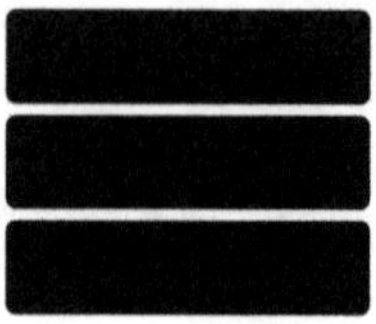

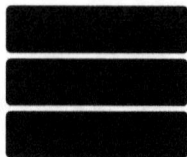

The Lion is associated with the Qian trigram. Qian is *spirit force,* or Heaven, and the father of the trigrams. Qian is pure Yang and represents strength and creativity. In the body it represents the head, and the Interlocking Palm in the martial arts.

To perform the Lion, walk the circle in the Holding The Spear Standing Palm and perform a Single Palm Change. When exiting the Single Palm Change, however, the right hand will slide out under the left elbow as the left hand turns over to assume its position at the forehead.

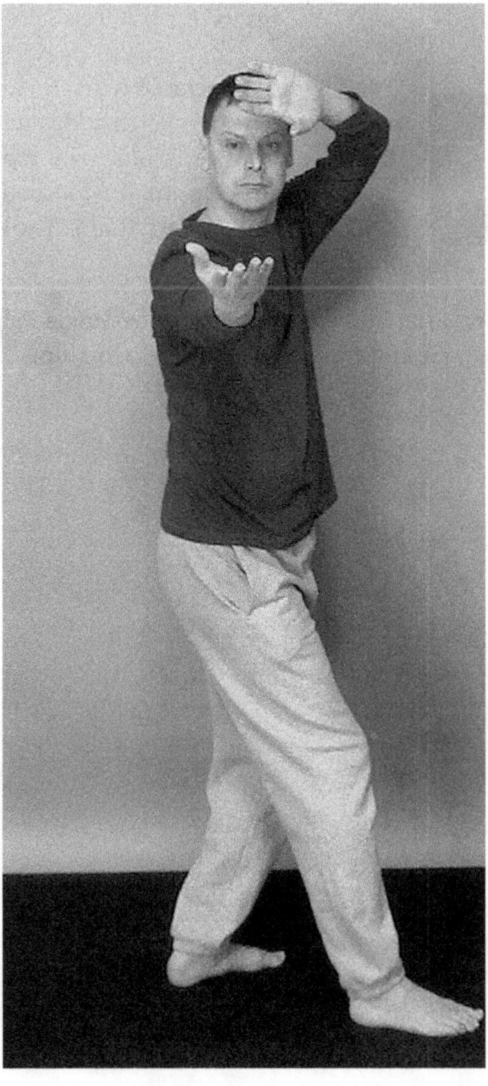

Lion

QILIN

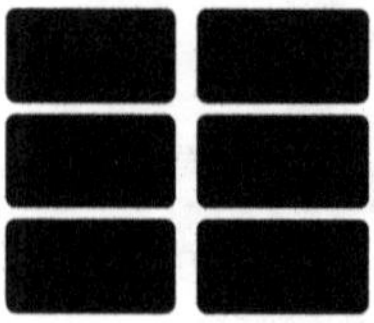

The Qilin is associated with the Kun trigram. Kun represents the Earth and is the mother of the trigrams. Kun is pure Yin, represents the receptive and service. In the body it is the belly, and in the martial arts it is the Returning Palm.

Begin with the initial toe-in step of the Single Palm Change, but turn the left hand over so the palm is facing up.

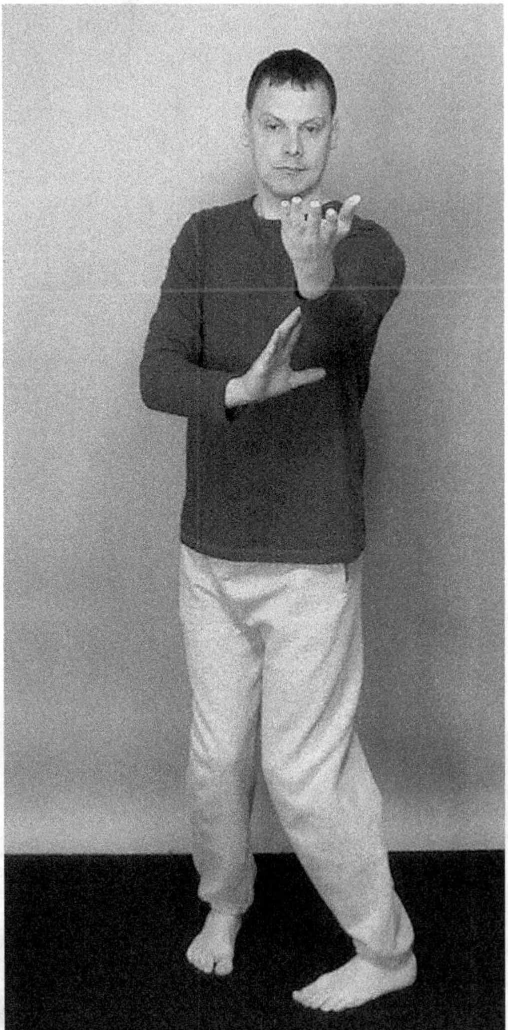

Qilin - One

Continue with a toe-out step of the left foot. The right hand begins to travel under the left elbow as you make this turn.

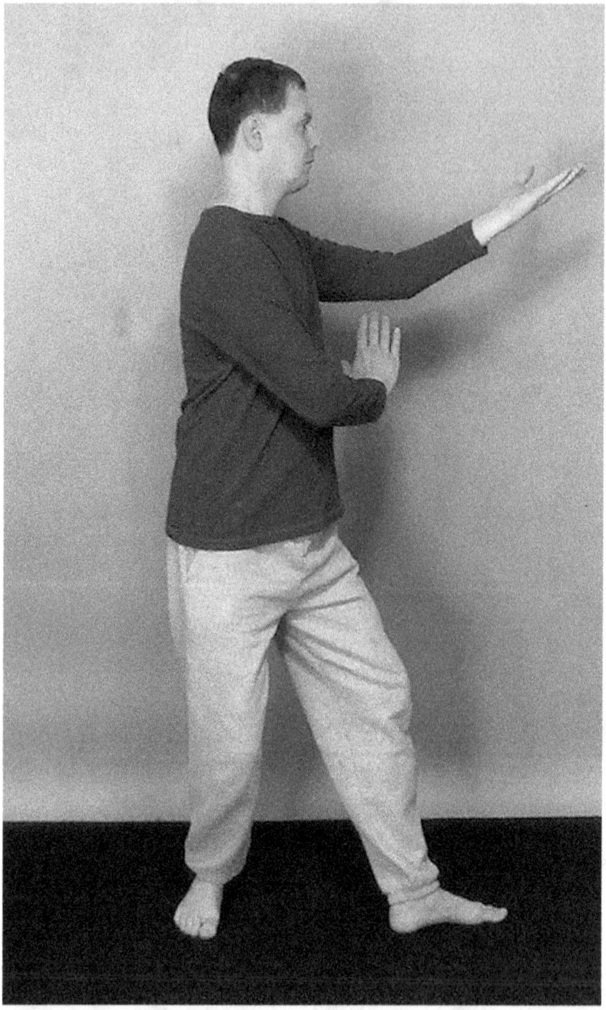

Qilin - Two

Toe-in with the right foot while maintaining the position of the left hand. The right hand slides under the elbow of the left arm.

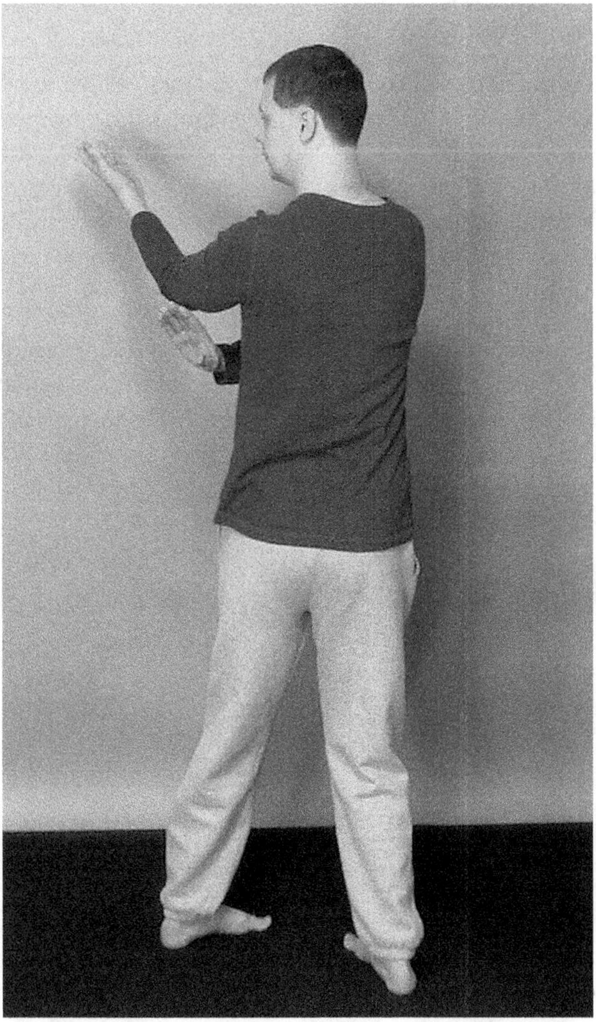

Qilin - Three

Perform a large toe-out with the left foot so the that the heel of the foot is opposite the heel of the right foot. The hand positions do not change; maintain focus on the fingers of the left hand.

Bring the right foot next to the left foot, but do not put it down on the floor. It should be near the ankle of the left foot as in the Double Palm Change. Pull the right hand back down to the right side of the waist as you shrug with the left arm and shoulder. The pulling down of the right hand, the shrugging of the left arm, and the right foot arriving at the ankle of the left foot all happen simultaneously. All movement comes to a momentary stop.

After spinning rapidly through the previous postures this stop can cause you to lose your balance, so it is acceptable for beginners to drop the right foot momentarily to maintain balance. The goal is to be able to stop firmly on the fixed foot without becoming unbalanced.

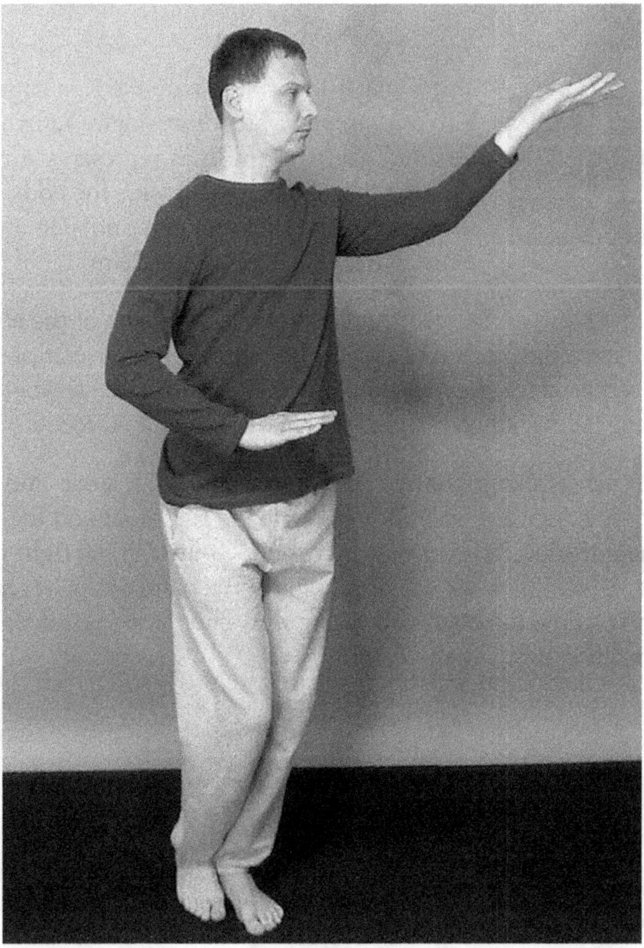

Qilin - Four

Without putting the right foot down on the floor, bring it around and toe-in with the right foot as you pierce the right hand past the left arm. The left arm wraps up and draws in as you toe-in. The posture is now like the closed form of Single Palm Change.

Complete a Single Palm Change and begin walking in the opposite direction.

SNAKE

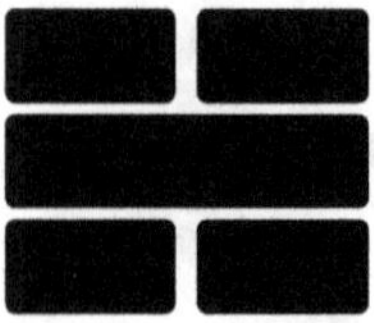

The Snake is associated with the Kan trigram. Kan represents water, the single Yang line between the two Yin lines represents a river running through a gorge. Inside the body, it is the kidneys and the ears on the outside. In the martial arts, it is the Flowing Palm.

The Flowing Palm Change turns to the outside of the circle. Because of this, you will not change direction after completing this sequence of movements, and will have to add a Single or Double Palm change to practice Snake in the other direction.

When walking counterclockwise around the circle and the left foot is forward, step forward with the right foot and toe-out, to the outside of the circle. When you toe-out with the right foot, bend the elbow of the left arm to bring the palm of the left hand even with the forehead and facing out. The right hand does not move, and guards the side of the body.

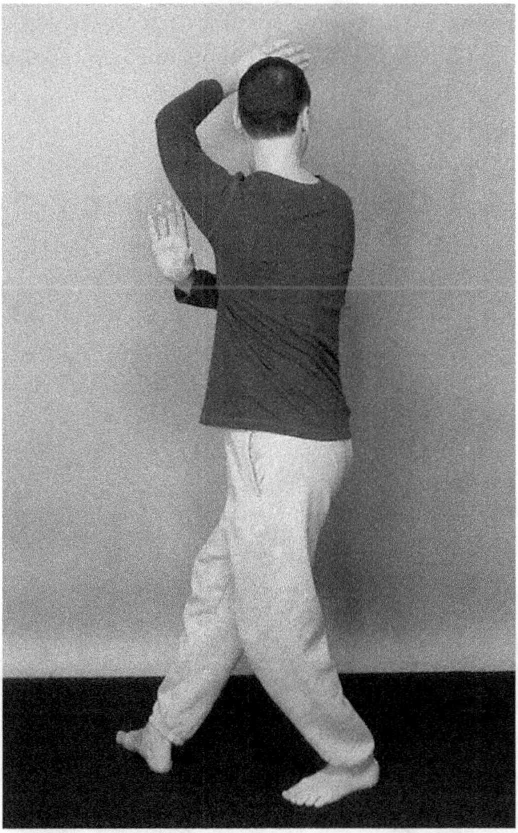

Snake - One

Toe-in with the left foot, creating a large sweep across the floor. The hand positions remain the same, but the large toe-in movement causes the torso to twist so it is facing in the opposite direction, and the left hand to pierce above the forehead with palm facing up.

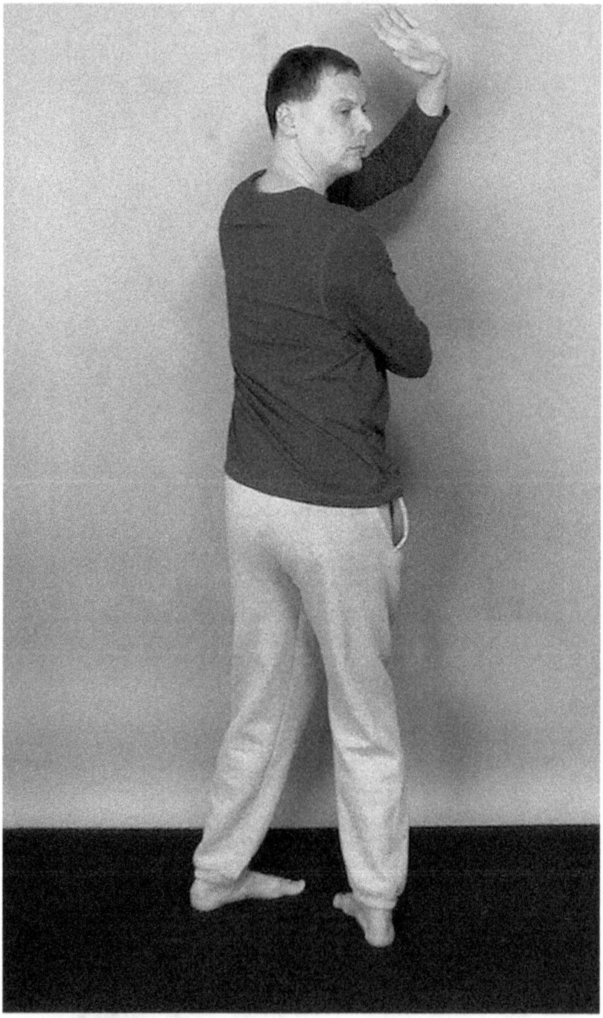

Snake - Two

Perform a large toe-out with the right foot so the right heel is opposite the left heel. The toes of the right foot are pointing forward along the line of the circle. This is similar to the lowering posture of Double Palm Change, but more weight is on the back leg.

Complete the Flowing Palm Change by turning the right foot out on its heel, then toe-in with the left foot to perform a Single Palm Change. When you have completed that change, you will be walking in the same direction.

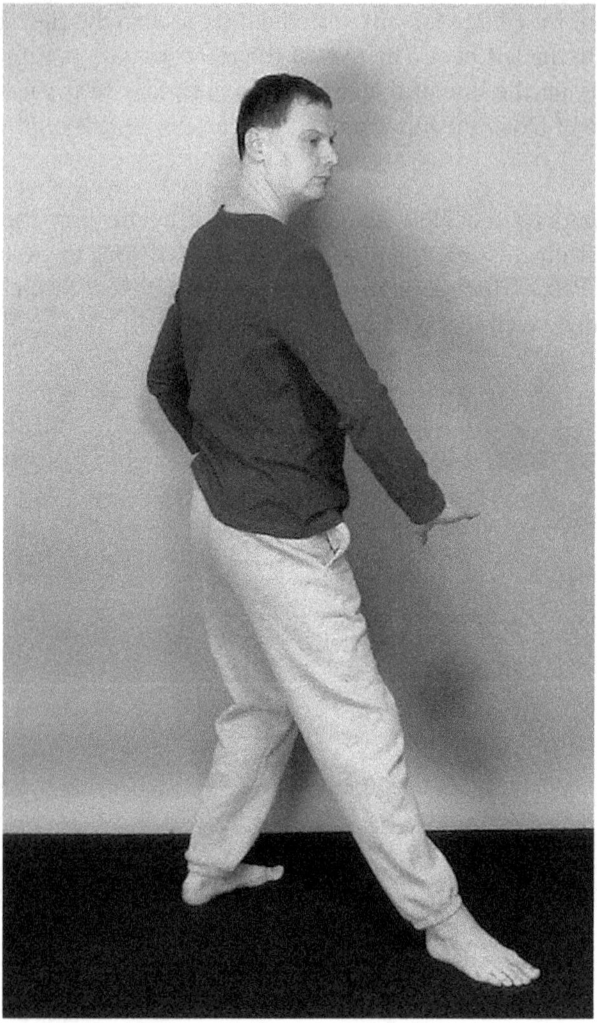

Snake - Three

SPARROW HAWK

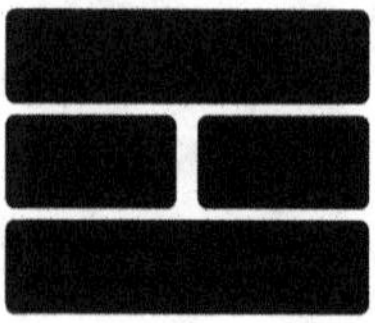

The Sparrow Hawk is associated with the Li trigram. Li represents Fire, the single Yin line between the two Yang lines represents the radiance of a fire burning. Li is visualizing and represents the eyes on the outside of the body and the heart on the inside. In the martial arts, it is the Lying palm.

From the left Pushing Millstone Palm toe-in with the right foot to begin the change.

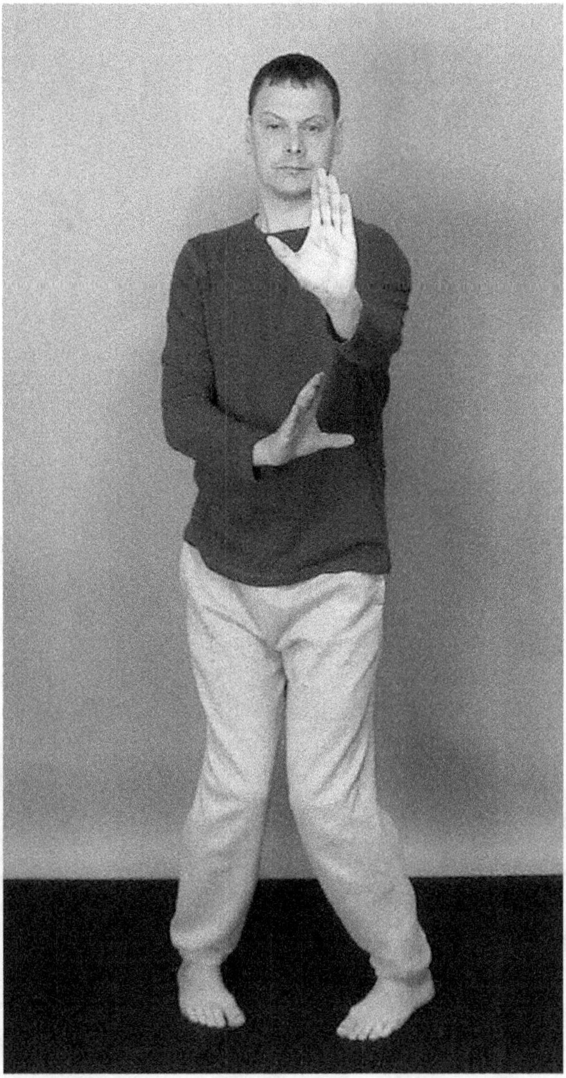

Sparrow Hawk -- One

Toe-out with the left foot and turn the palms over so they are pushing in the direction of the change.

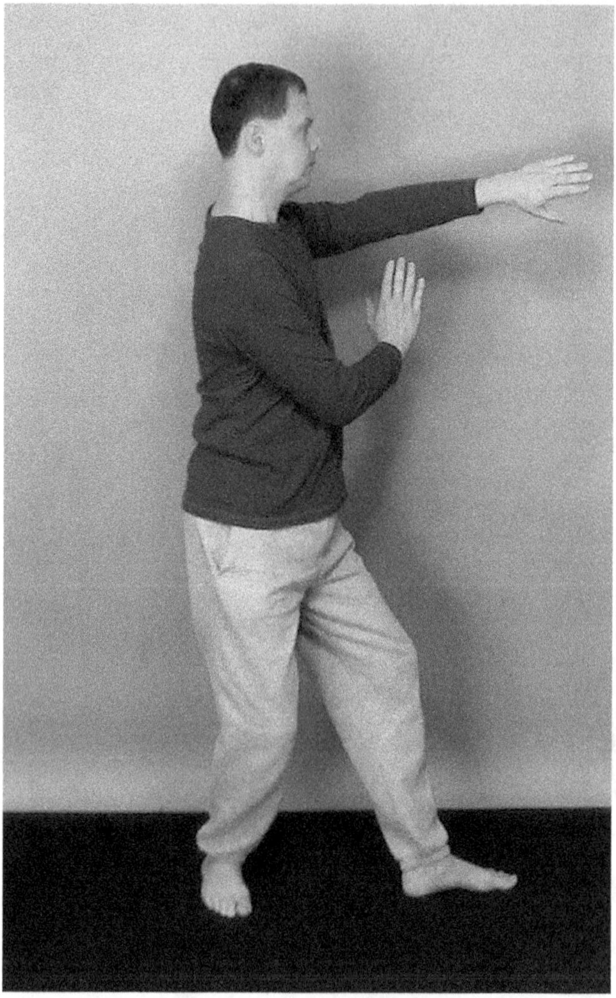

Sparrow Hawk -- Two

When you toe-in, do not pierce the right hand past the left arm, rather turn the right palm out as in the Sky and Ground Palm posture. The feeling should be like the right arm is pushing against something solid, causing the lower part of your spring to get stuck while the upper part continues to load for a strike.

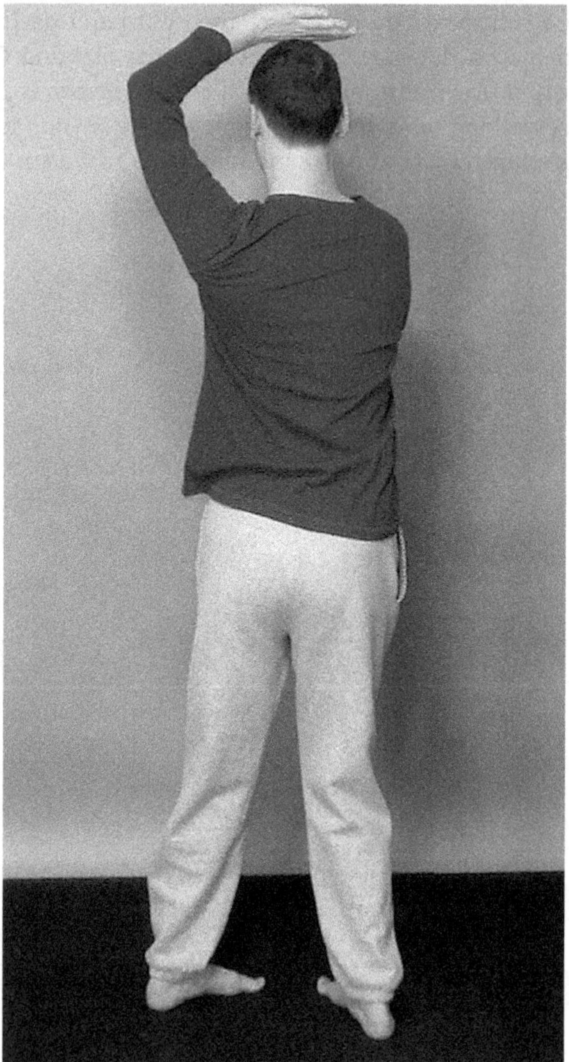

Sparrow Hawk -- Three

The left hand does not remain fixed as in the Single Palm Change, rather it turns palm up, above the head, preparing to perform an arcing chop with next movement.

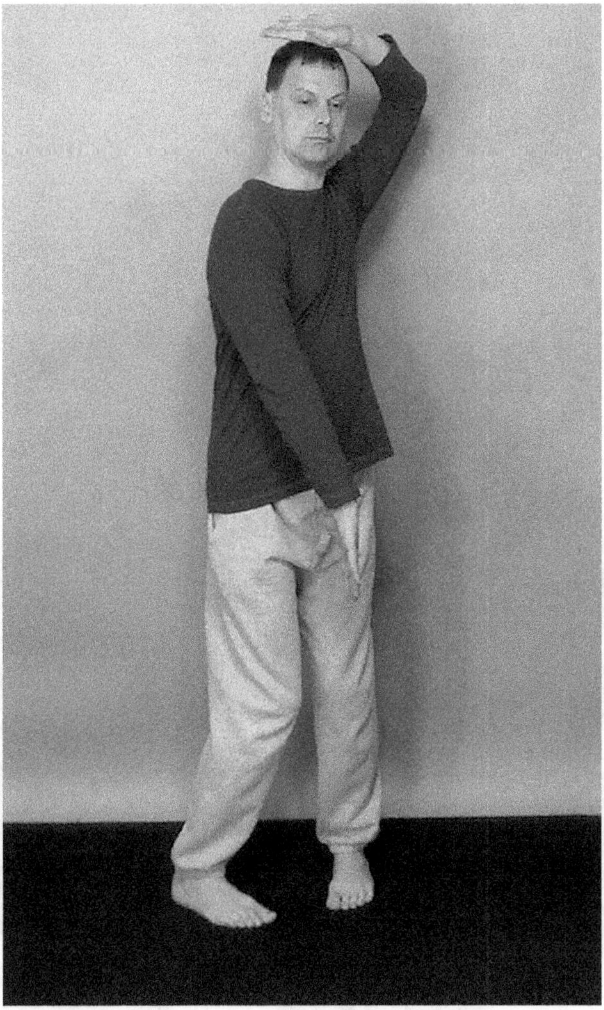

Sparrow Hawk -- Three (front)

Spin on the toes of the right foot as in the Double Palm Change and bring the left hand and left leg around in two arcs. The left hand performs a chop across the head and neck of your opponent while the left knee comes up to strike their lower body.

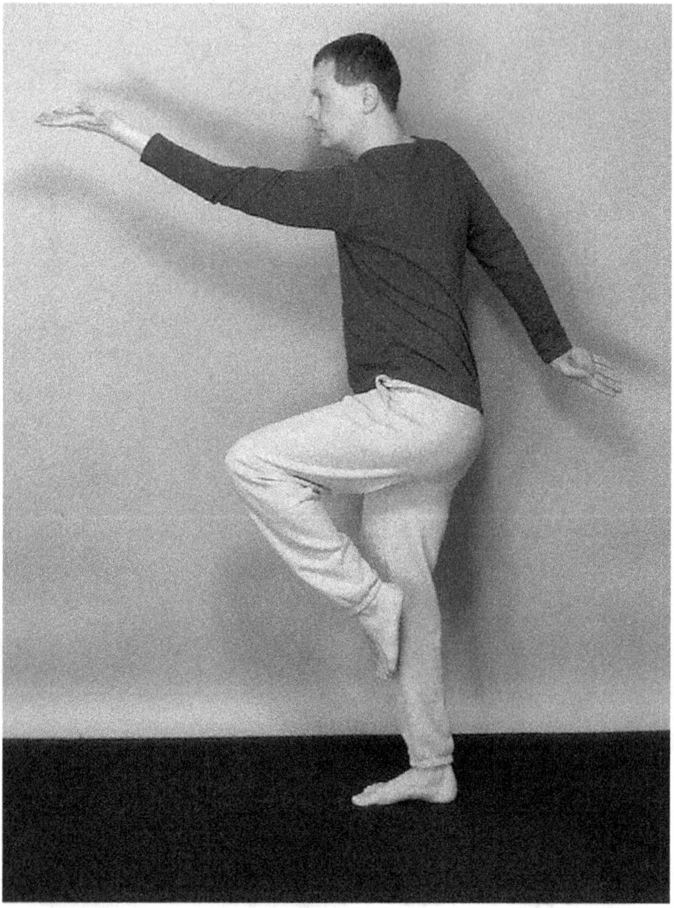

Sparrow Hawk -- Four

From this posture, lower the left leg and foot into a large toe-out posture along the edge of the circle. Then perform a large sweep of the right leg as you toe-in for a Single Palm Change to end the form.

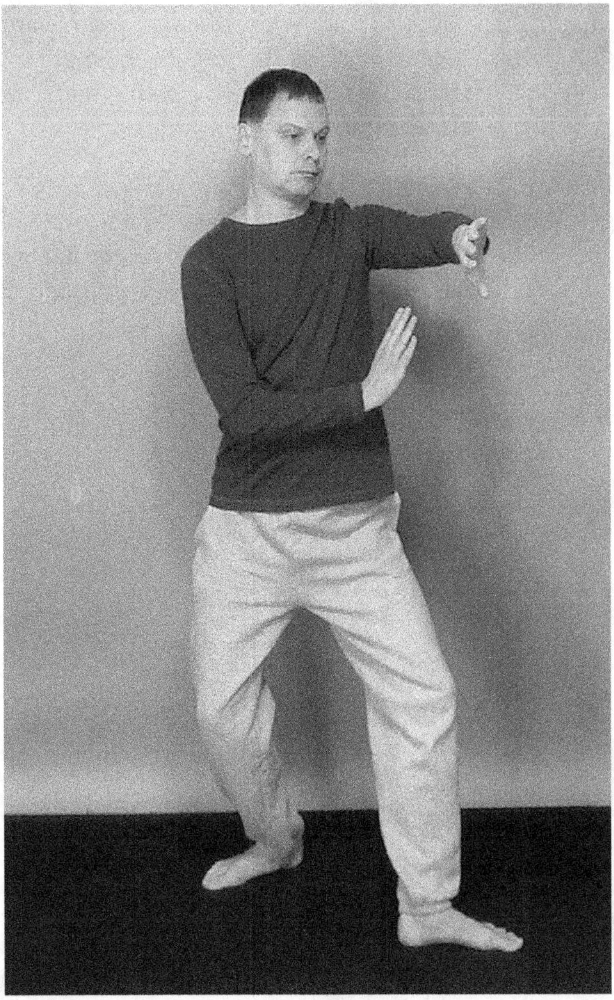

Sparrow Hawk -- Five

DRAGON

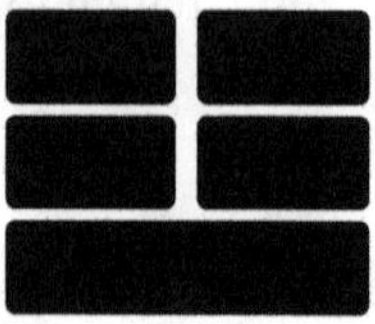

The Dragon is associated with the Zhen trigram. Zhen represents Thunder, the two Yin lines above the single Yang line represent clouds building for a storm. Zhen is arousing and represents the feet. In the martial arts it represents the left side of the body and the Upholding palm.

The Dragon is the Supporting Palm with a Single Palm Change. As you exit Single Palm Change, do not put your left hand inside the elbow of the right arm. The right hand comes out under the left arm as the left palm turns over to face down. Hold an imaginary ball with the hands.

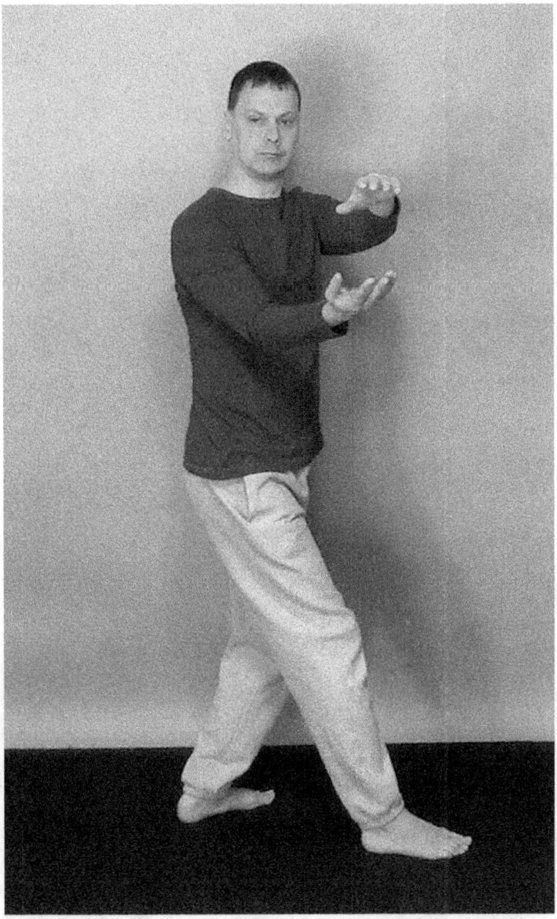

Dragon -- One

Spread your arms like the wings of a Dragon taking flight. Steal a Step with the right foot, Sweep Step with the left foot and

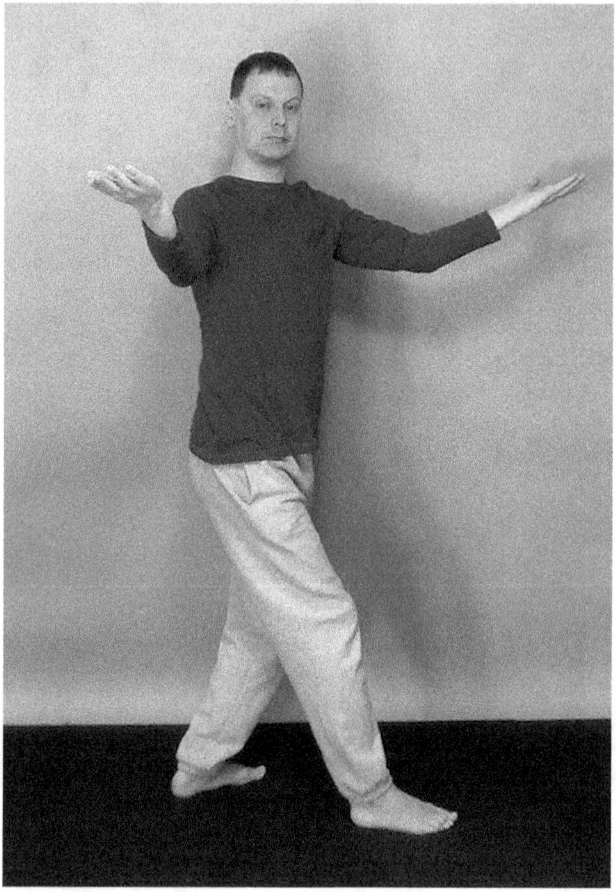

Dragon -- Two

walk in the clockwise direction.

BEAR

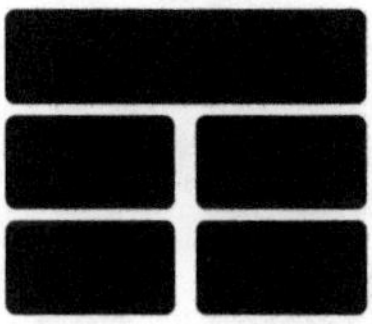

The Bear is associated with the Gen trigram. Gen represents a Mountain, the two Yin lines below the single Yang line represent a mountain reaching into the clouds. Gen is bound and represents stillness. In the body it is the hands. In the martial arts it is represented by the upper back and Behind the Body palm.

The Bear is another variation on the Single Palm Change with a thrust from under your chin to strike your opponent. From the left Pushing Millstone Palm toe-in with the right foot to begin the change.

Toe-out with the left foot and turn the palms over so they are pushing in the direction of the change.

When you toe-in do not pierce the right palm past the left arm, rather curl its fingers together and bring it next to your right hip. Pull the left hand up and under your chin so the fingers are pointing straight out and the elbow is against your body.

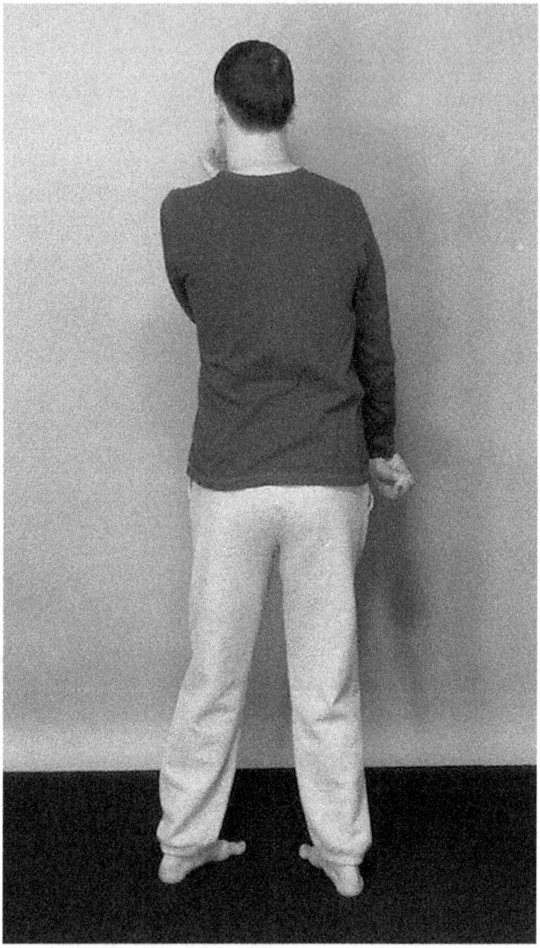

Bear -- One

Do not toe-out, instead pierce out with the hand from under your chin and push back with the right palm, curling the fingers into a pecking hand form. As you do this raise the left leg and strike up with the knee.

Conclude by lowering the raised leg into a large toe-out position and perform a Single Palm Change as you did in the Sparrow Hawk.

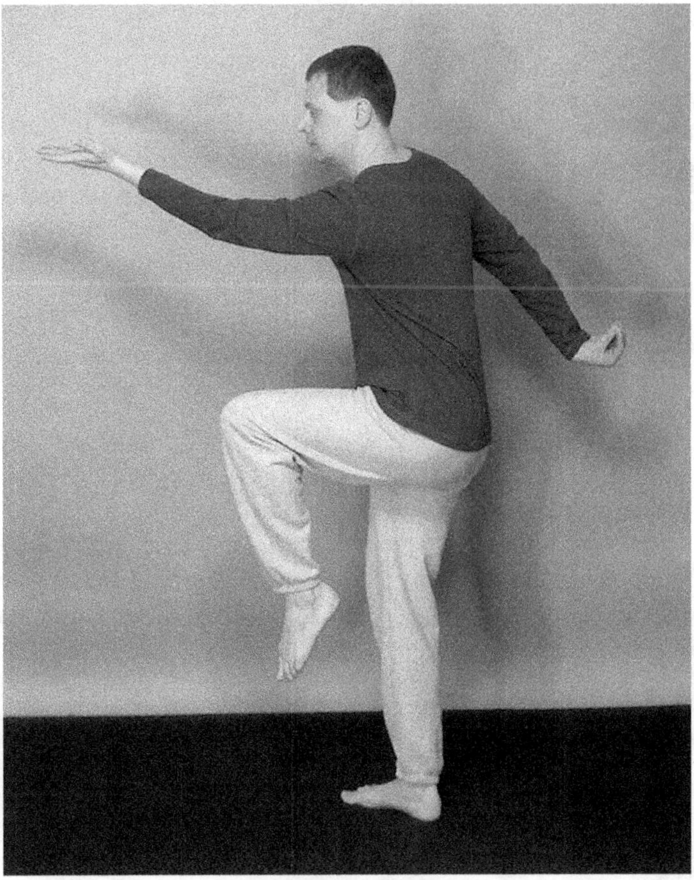

Bear -- Two

PHOENIX

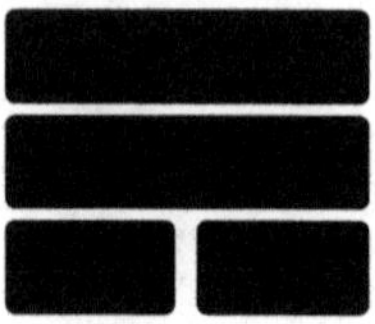

The Phoenix is associated with the Sun trigram. Sun represents the wind, the single Yin line below the double Yang line representing movement under heaven. Sun is associated with wood. It represents the limbs and lower back in the body, and the Windmill, or Hurricane Palm, in the martial arts.

The Phoenix is Rolling the Ball Palm with a unique rolling the ball palm change.

Toe-in with the right foot as if beginning a Single Palm Change. Do not change the hand positions.

Toe-out with the left foot and move the right hand in an arc from above the head down to waist level. This is similar to the movement you practiced when doing a Simple Change from this posture.

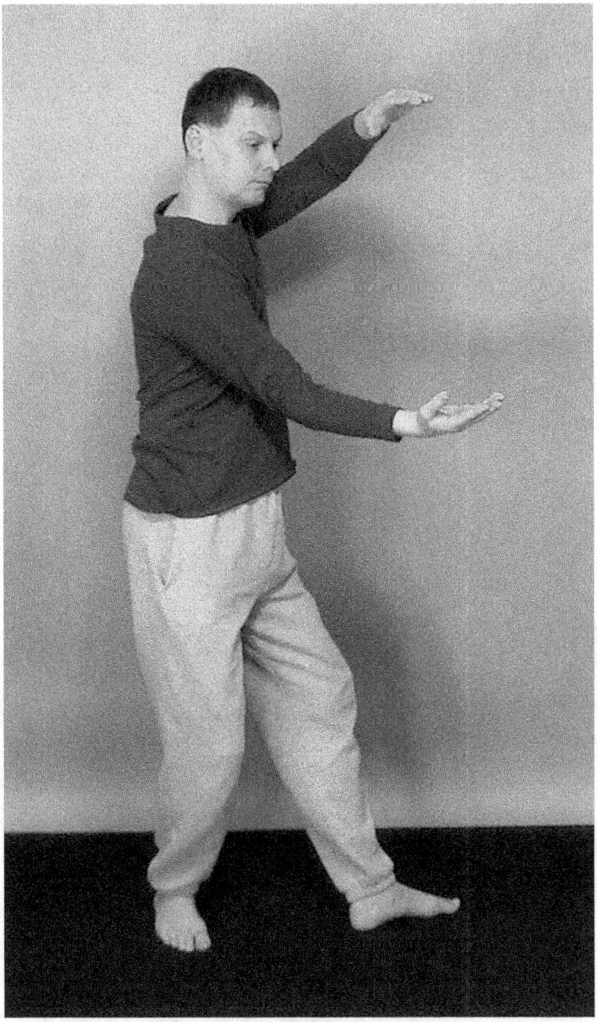

Phoenix -- One

Toe-in with the right foot and exchange the hand positions again. The right hand moves in an arc above the head. Both hands should move as if they are holding a large ball, and rolling it about the body.

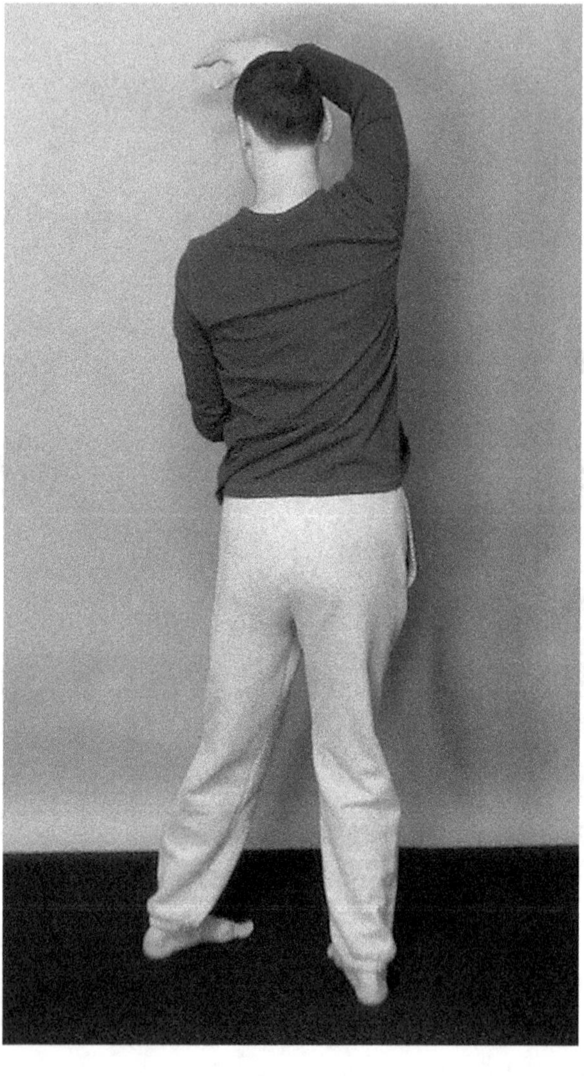

Phoenix -- Two

Perform a large toe-out with the left foot. As you toe-out bring the arms down with both palms facing up, as if you are now cradling the ball against your chest.

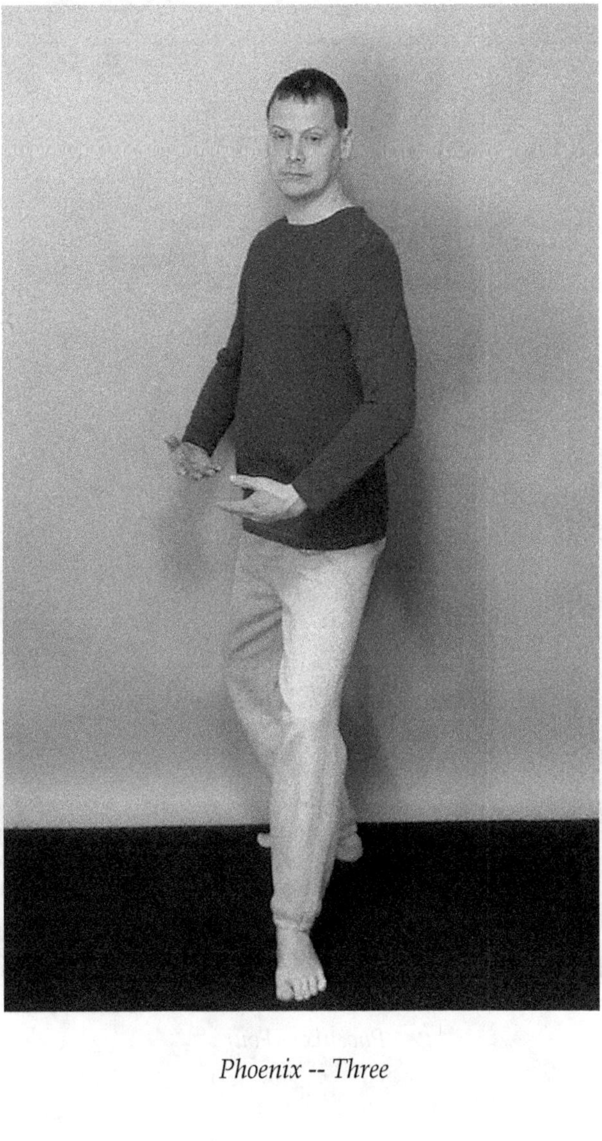

Phoenix -- Three

Turn the left foot out on its heel and toe-in again with the right foot to perform a Single Palm Change. As you exit the Single Palm Change assume Rolling the Ball Palm in the clockwise direction.

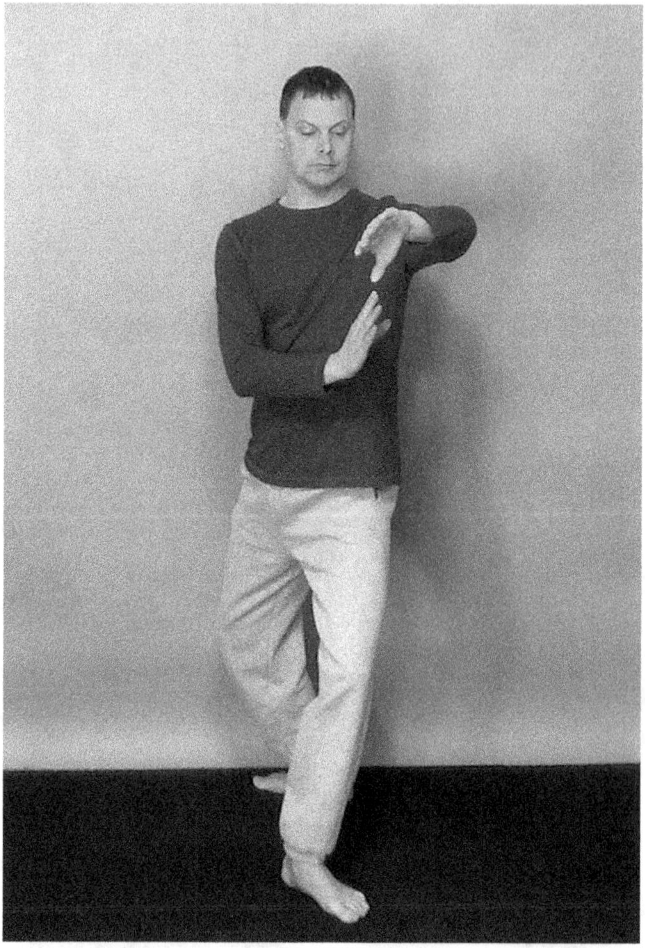

Phoenix -- Four

MONKEY

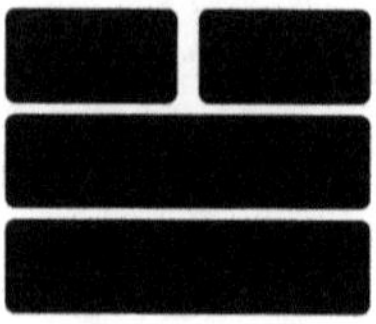

The Monkey is associated with the Dui trigram. Dui is a marsh or lake, the single Yin line above the double Yang lines representing water lying on the earth. Dui represents the mouth in the body. In the martial arts it is the Embracing palm and the right side of the waist.

You are already familiar with the Monkey, it is the Holding The Fruit Palm with a Single Palm Change. When you exit the Single Palm Change bring both hands together into Holding The Fruit Palm.

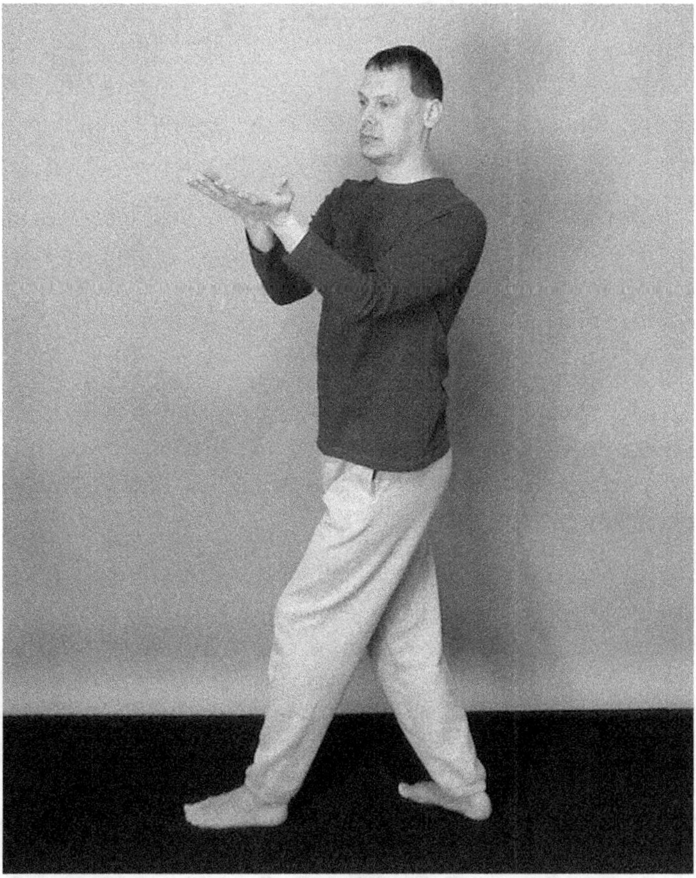

Monkey

RECOMMENDED PRACTICE

You now have all the tools you need for a lifetime of healthy practice. Taking advantage of these tools, and using them regularly is a responsibility you must take seriously.

In the next section I present the Supplemental Exercises as a complete set that you should perform daily. If getting a piece of the day for yourself is still an issue, then you can use the exercise routine in that section as an excuse for needing that time.

Baguazhang allows you to practice the most basic and beneficial of exercises--walking--in a limited amount of space with a limitless potential for variety. If you find that your practice is becoming stale you can learn more changes or modify the ones you already know.

The American Heart Association recommends using a pedometer to count the steps you take in a day. From this measurement, you can determine how active or sedentary your lifestyle is. Armed with this information you can develop a plan to improve your general health.

Use this chart as a reference:

ACTIVITY LEVEL	NUMBER OF STEPS
Sedentary	less than 5,000
Low	5,000 - 7,500
Moderate	7,500 - 10,000
Active	10,000 or more

10,000 steps is a long way, about 5 miles, and it is unlikely that you can walk 5 miles of circles in a single session, or that you would keep that pace up for very long.

At ten steps a circle you need 1000 circles--500 clockwise and 500 counterclockwise to reach 10,000 steps. That is 25 circles in each direction for each posture in this book.

I have walked 1000 circles on days when my spirit would not let me do anything else. I have a large repertoire of changes that I put into my practice during such sessions. Usually, this involves my trying changes normally taught from the Pushing Millstone Palm with another Standing Palm. I have never walked 1000 circles in a single session, however.

If you plan to walk 1000 circles in a day then I encourage you to try the Single Palm Change, Double Palm Change, Qilin, Snake, Sparrow Hawk, Bear, and Phoenix changes from Standing Palms other than Pushing Millstone Palm. Have fun with your practice.

It is unlikely that you could perform all the exercises in this book everyday, you simply do not have that much time. Here are some recommendations to help you make the most of your limited practice time.

- Ideally, practice for one hour every day. After you have learned the Internal Power Set you should be able to complete it in about 20 minutes. Practice a combination of circle walking and standing postures for the remainder of the hour; with the emphasis on walking.

- If you do not have an uninterrupted hour in your day, then practice the Internal Power Set early in the day and circle walk later in the day.

- Walk at least three circles in each of the Standing Palms before you choose one of the postures from the Eight Trigram section to focus on for the remainder of your practice.

- Once a week, go crazy, and mix up a wide variety of changes and postures changing from one to another each time you change directions on the circle. Do not worry about proper form or function; have fun.

• Once a week, use Sliding Step or Pole Step with each of the Standing Palm postures. Concentrate on your breathing and proper body alignment.

• If you are traveling and do not have space to perform the circle walking practice, then practice the standing postures. Note that you do not want to put your face onto a hotel room floor, they are not very clean. Therefore, you can skip the Internal Power Set for an hour of standing practice. Walk around your hotel room between standing sessions; do not sit down until you have completed your practice.

• When you return home, practice the Internal Power Set immediately, it is a great way to recover from travel stiffness and reminds you to get back into your routine.

• If you find yourself lying about in front of the television, try practicing the standing postures during commercial breaks. Choose one posture for each commercial break, and hold it until the break is over. I understand that this violates the *meditation* component I discussed in the Attention section, but it is better than lying around.

• Try to spend at least 10 minutes in standing practice before you go to bed at night. It will clear your head and help with sleep.

• If you can get outside to perform your circle walking practice, then you should do so. If a neighbor or passerby asks what you are doing, recommend this book and direct them to The Walking Circle web site to buy it. (http://www.thewalkingcircle.com).

THE INTERNAL POWER SET

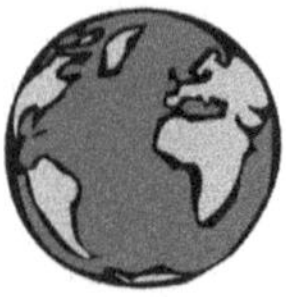

In classical internal martial art practice, there are several Qigong sets designed to teach *internal power.* They are composed of stretching, massage, and breathing exercises designed to develop or transport Qi throughout the body.

As I related at the beginning of this book, there was not enough movement in those exercises to prevent my hip pain. From that pain, however, a pearl developed. My pain forced me to explore outside traditional internal martial art routines to improve my physical fitness. From that exploration I developed the following Internal Power routine.

I developed this routine from a line in a Taijiquan classic text that says: "Power is generated by the feet, transferred through the legs, directed by the waist, and transmitted through the arms to the hands."

Perform the supplemental exercises in this order. Descriptions of the exercises are at the corresponding page number.

EXERCISE	PAGE
Arm Circles	62
Butterfly Front	67
The Turtle	99
Back Kick	100
Push Up	62
The Bellows	79
Bridge	84
Hurdlers Stretch	86
Forward Bend	87
Floor Twist	128
Butterfly Back	68
Foot Circles	98
Hip Lift	69
Crunches	131
Horse Posture	58

APPENDIX

CHINESE DYNASTIES

This table lists the Chinese Dynasties from the early Zho to the Qin. Significant events from world history are listed in the far right column for perspective.

DYNASTY	SIGNIFICANCE	PERSPECTIVE
Zho (1122 - 255 BCE)	King Wen of Zhou (1099 - 1050 BCE). Laozi (590 - 500 BCE). Gautama Buddha (563 - 483 BCE). Confucius (551 - 479 BCE).	David is King of Israel (1006 BCE).
Qin (221 - 206 BCE)	The Birth of China.	Hannibal defeats the Romans at Cannae (216 BCE).
Han (206 BCE - 220 CE)	Confucianism adopted as state creed.	Julius Caesar, Rome (100 - 44 BCE). Crucifixion of Christ (33 CE).
Period of Disunion (265 - 581 CE)	Bodhidharma (440 - 534) Shaolin temple (495). Bodhidarma in China (520). Creation of Zen Buddhism (527).	The sacking of Rome by the Visigoths (410).
Sui, Tang Dynasties (581 - 908 CE)	Buddhism adopted as state creed. Imperial examinations for Confucian scholars. *Journey to the West.*	Koran written (650). Charlemagne's Holy Roman Empire (742 - 814).
Song Dynasty (960 - 1279 CE)	Zhang Sanfeng (1247 - 1370) creates Taijiquan.	Magna Carta signed in England (1215).
Yuan (1279 - 1368 CE)	Construction of Beijing and The Forbidden City is begun.	Black Death in Europe (1347 - 1351)

DYNASTY	SIGNIFICANCE	PERSPECTIVE
Ming (1368 - 1644 CE)	*Ming* porcelain reaches Europe and becomes known as *China*. Portuguese colonize Macao (1557).	Columbus sails to America (1492). Shakespeare born (1564).
Qing (1644 - 1912 CE)	Dong Haichuan (1797 - 1882). Yin Fu (1840 - 1909). Cheng Ting Hua (1848 - 1900).	US Declaration of Independence (1776). Communist manifesto is printed (1848). American Civil War (1861).
Republican Era (1912 - 1949 CE)	Sun Lu Tang (1861 - 1932).	World War I (1914). World War II (1939).

APPENDIX

FIVE PHASES ASSOCIATIONS

These tables list associations of The Five Phases. These associations are attributed to the Yellow Emperor and the *Huangdi Neijing*.

WOOD

CONCEPT	ASSOCIATION
DIRECTION	East
SEASON	Spring
WEATHER	Wind
PLANET	Jupiter
NUMEROLOGY	3 + 5 = 8
NATURAL ELEMENT	Grass
ANIMAL	Chicken
CEREAL OR GRAIN	Wheat
MUSICAL NOTE	Lute
COLOR	Green
FLAVOR	Sour
SMELL	Urine
ZHANG ORGAN (YIN)	Liver
FU ORGAN (YANG)	Gall Bladder
ORIFICE	Eyes
BODY PART	Tendon/Ligaments
SOUND	Shout
EMOTION	Anger
PATHOLOGICAL FUNCTION	Clench Fist/Spasm
LOCATION	Neck/Head

CONCEPT	ASSOCIATION
SPIRIT	Soul

FIRE

CONCEPT	ASSOCIATION
DIRECTION	South
SEASON	Summer
WEATHER	Heat
PLANET	Mars
NUMEROLOGY	2 + 5 = 7
NATURAL ELEMENT	Fire
ANIMAL	Goat
CEREAL OR GRAIN	Corn
MUSICAL NOTE	Pipe Organ
COLOR	Red
FLAVOR	Bitter
SMELL	Scorched
ZHANG ORGAN (YIN)	Heart
FU ORGAN (YANG)	Small Intestine
ORIFICE	Ear
BODY PART	Vessels
SOUND	Laughter
EMOTION	Joy
PATHOLOGICAL FUNCTION	Anxious Look
LOCATION	Chest/Ribs

CONCEPT	ASSOCIATION
SPIRIT	Spirit

EARTH

CONCEPT	ASSOCIATION
DIRECTION	Central
SEASON	Late Summer
WEATHER	Damp
PLANET	Saturn
NUMEROLOGY	5
NATURAL ELEMENT	Earth
ANIMAL	Cow
CEREAL OR GRAIN	Rye
MUSICAL NOTE	Drum
COLOR	Yellow
FLAVOR	Sweet
SMELL	Fragrant
ZHANG ORGAN (YIN)	Spleen
FU ORGAN (YANG)	Stomach
ORIFICE	Mouth
BODY PART	Muscles/Flesh
SOUND	Singing
EMOTION	Distress/Worry
PATHOLOGICAL FUNC-TION	Spitting
LOCATION	Midback

CONCEPT	ASSOCIATION
SPIRIT	Logic

METAL

CONCEPT	ASSOCIATION
DIRECTION	West
SEASON	Autumn
WEATHER	Dryness
PLANET	Venus
NUMEROLOGY	4 + 5 = 9
NATURAL ELEMENT	Metal
ANIMAL	Hore
CEREAL OR GRAIN	Rice
MUSICAL NOTE	Resonant
COLOR	White
FLAVOR	Pungent
SMELL	Fishy
ZHANG ORGAN (YIN)	Lung
FU ORGAN (YANG)	Large Intestine
ORIFICE	Nose
BODY PART	Skin/Hair
SOUND	Crying
EMOTION	Grief/Sadness
PATHOLOGICAL FUNCTION	Cough
LOCATION	Shoulder/Upper Back

CONCEPT	ASSOCIATION
SPIRIT	Courage

WATER

CONCEPT	ASSOCIATION
DIRECTION	North
SEASON	Winter
WEATHER	Cold
PLANET	Mercury
NUMEROLOGY	1 + 5 = 6
NATURAL ELEMENT	Water
ANIMAL	Pig
CEREAL OR GRAIN	Bean
MUSICAL NOTE	Stringed
COLOR	Black
FLAVOR	Salty
SMELL	Rotten
ZHANG ORGAN (YIN)	Kidney
FU ORGAN (YANG)	Bladder
ORIFICE	Anus/Urethra
BODY PART	Bones/Marrow
SOUND	Moaning
EMOTION	Fear
PATHOLOGICAL FUNCTION	Shivering
LOCATION	Low Back/Hips/Limbs

CONCEPT	ASSOCIATION
SPIRIT	Will

APPENDIX

FIVE PHASES DIAGRAM

This diagram illustrates the promoting and destroying aspects of the Five Phases.

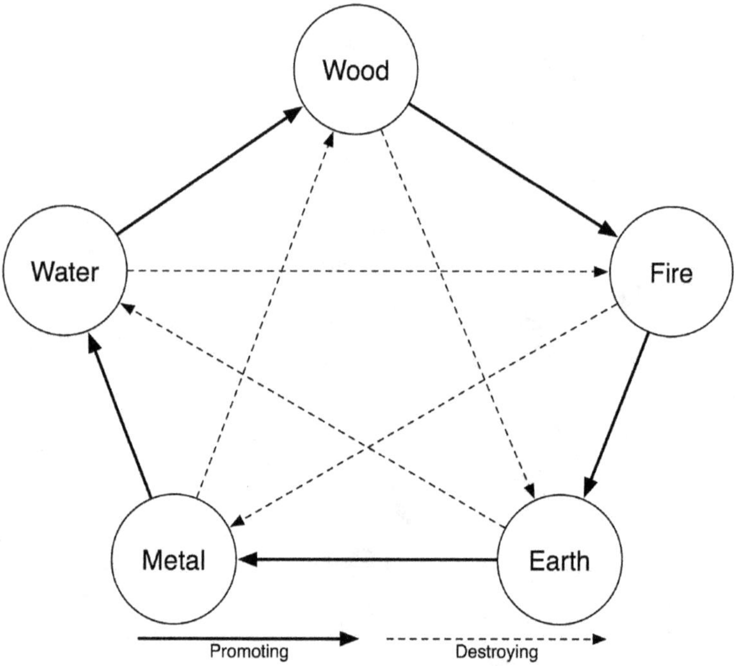

APPENDIX

TRIGRAM ASSOCIATIONS

These tables list a wide range of associations to the trigrams of the Bagua. These associations have developed over time, but most of them are attributed to either Ken Wen of the Zhou Dynasty or Confucius.

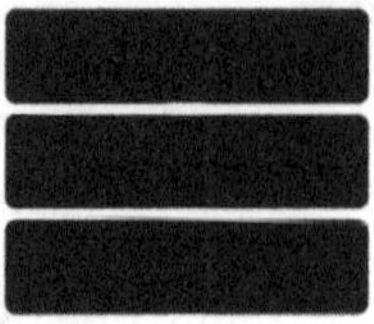

CONCEPT	ASSOCIATION
CHINESE NAME	Qian
IMAGE	Force, Heaven
PRE-HEAVEN BODY	Head
POST-HEAVEN BODY	Head
PRE-HEAVEN ANIMAL	Horse
POST-HEAVEN ANIMAL	Lion
FAMILY	Father
PERSONALITY	Creative
SEASON	Summer
PRE-HEAVEN DIRECTION	South
POST-HEAVEN DIRECTION	Northwest
MARTIAL FORM	Interlocking

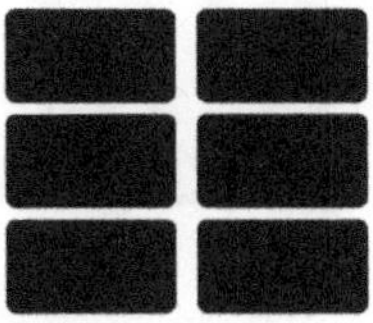

CONCEPT	ASSOCIATION
CHINESE NAME	Kun
IMAGE	Field, Earth
PRE-HEAVEN BODY	Belly
POST-HEAVEN BODY	Belly
PRE-HEAVEN ANIMAL	Ox
POST-HEAVEN ANIMAL	Qilin
FAMILY	Mother
PERSONALITY	Receptive
SEASON	Winter
PRE-HEAVEN DIRECTION	North
POST-HEAVEN DIRECTION	Southwest
MARTIAL FORM	Returning

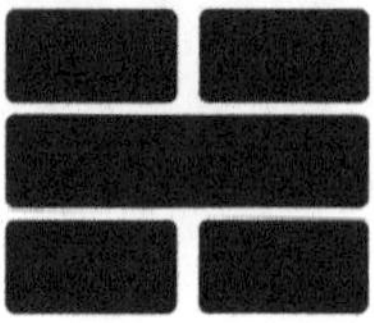

CONCEPT	ASSOCIATION
CHINESE NAME	Kan
IMAGE	Gorge, Stream
PRE-HEAVEN BODY	Ears
POST-HEAVEN BODY	Kidneys
PRE-HEAVEN ANIMAL	Pig
POST-HEAVEN ANIMAL	Snake
FAMILY	Middle Son
PERSONALITY	Toiling
SEASON	Fall
PRE-HEAVEN DIRECTION	West
POST-HEAVEN DIRECTION	North
MARTIAL FORM	Flowing

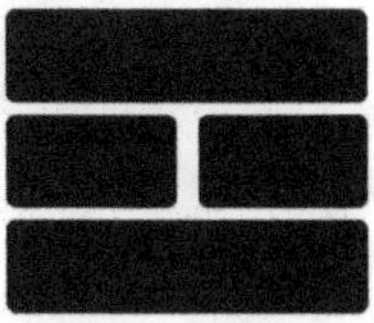

CONCEPT	ASSOCIATION
CHINESE NAME	Li
IMAGE	Radiance, Fire
PRE-HEAVEN BODY	Eyes
POST-HEAVEN BODY	Heart
PRE-HEAVEN ANIMAL	Pheasant
POST-HEAVEN ANIMAL	Sparrow Hawk
FAMILY	Middle Daughter
PERSONALITY	Visualizing
SEASON	Spring
PRE-HEAVEN DIRECTION	East
POST-HEAVEN DIRECTION	South
MARTIAL FORM	Lying

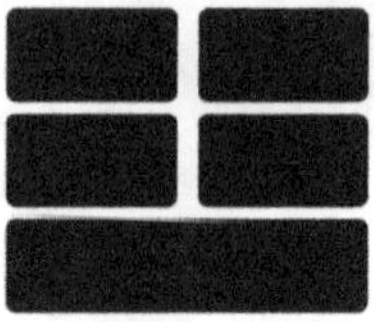

CONCEPT	ASSOCIATION
CHINESE NAME	Zhen
IMAGE	Shake, Thunder
PRE-HEAVEN BODY	Feet
POST-HEAVEN BODY	Left Waist
PRE-HEAVEN ANIMAL	Dragon
POST-HEAVEN ANIMAL	Dragon
FAMILY	Eldest Son
PERSONALITY	Arousing
SEASON	Winter
PRE-HEAVEN DIRECTION	Northeast
POST-HEAVEN DIRECTION	East
MARTIAL FORM	Upholding

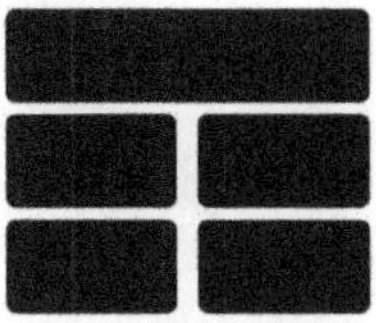

CONCEPT	ASSOCIATION
CHINESE NAME	Gen
IMAGE	Bound, Mountain
PRE-HEAVEN BODY	Hands
POST-HEAVEN BODY	Upper Back
PRE-HEAVEN ANIMAL	Dog
POST-HEAVEN ANIMAL	Bear
FAMILY	Youngest Son
PERSONALITY	Accomplishing
SEASON	Fall
PRE-HEAVEN DIRECTION	Northwest
POST-HEAVEN DIRECTION	Northeast
MARTIAL FORM	Behind the Body

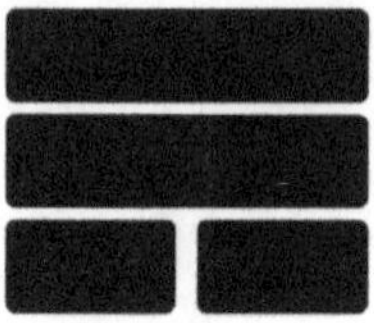

CONCEPT	ASSOCIATION
CHINESE NAME	Sun
IMAGE	Ground, Wind, Wood
PRE-HEAVEN BODY	Limbs
POST-HEAVEN BODY	Lower Back
PRE-HEAVEN ANIMAL	Chicken
POST-HEAVEN ANIMAL	Fenghuang
FAMILY	Eldest Daughter
PERSONALITY	Gentle
SEASON	Summer
PRE-HEAVEN DIRECTION	Southwest
POST-HEAVEN DIRECTION	Southeast
MARTIAL FORM	Windmill

CONCEPT	ASSOCIATION
CHINESE NAME	Dui
IMAGE	Open, Marsh, Lake
PRE-HEAVEN BODY	Mouth
POST-HEAVEN BODY	Right Waist
PRE-HEAVEN ANIMAL	Sheep
POST-HEAVEN ANIMAL	Monkey
FAMILY	Youngest Daughter
PERSONALITY	Stimulating
SEASON	Spring
PRE-HEAVEN DIRECTION	Southest
POST-HEAVEN DIRECTION	West
MARTIAL FORM	Embracing

APPENDIX

THREE INJURIES OF THE INNER SCHOOL

• Exerting Qi: Martial arts as physical exercise causing harm to the student is discussed in the Martial Arts section. Remember that according to Sun Lu Tang, Zhang Sanfeng recognized this overexertion and created Taijiquan.

• Clumsy Strength. Clumsy strength results when you overexert. There are many hints in this book on how to avoid the use of clumsy strength (*See* the Internal Harmonies in Trinity Posture section).

• Expanding the Breast, Raising the Abdomen: If the breast and abdomen are not sunk and relaxed (as described in the standing section), then you will be off balance, you will have to use too much strength, and you will overexert yourself in your practice.

SELECTED BIBLIOGRAPHY

Chaline, E. (2003). *The Book of Zen.* Hauppauge, New York: Barrons.

Deng, M.-D. (2006). *The Living I Ching.* San Francisco, California: Harper Collins.

Dr. Wang, S., & Dr. Liu, J. L. (1995). *Qi Gong for Health & Longevity: The Ancient Chinese Art of Relaxation, Meditation, Physical Fitness*. Tustin, California: The East Health Development Group.

Dr. Williams, T. (1996). *The Complete Illustrated Guide to Chinese Medicine: A Comprehensive System for Health and Fitness.* New York, New York: Barnes & Noble.

Dr. Yang, J.-M. (1991). *Advanced Yang Style Tai Chi Chuan Volume One Tai Chi Theory and Tai Chi Jing*. Jamaica Plain, Massachusetts: YMAA Publication Center.

Dr. Yang, J.-M. (1982). *Yang Style Tai Chi Chuan.* United States of America: Unique Publications, Inc.

Dr. Yang, J.-M. (1985). *Chi Kung Health & Martial Arts.* Jamaica Plain, Massachusetts: YMAA Publication Center.

Dr. Yang, J.-M. (2001). *Tai Chi Secrets of the Wu & Li Styles.* Boston Massachusetts: YMAA Publication Center.

Dr. Yang, J.-M. (1997). *Hsing Yi Chuan.* Jamaica Plain, Massachusetts: YMAA Publication Center.

Egoscue, P., & Gittines, R. (2000). *Pain Free: A Revolutionary Method For Stopping Chronic Pain.* New York, New York: Bantam Books.

Egoscue, P., & Gittines, R. (2001). *The Egoscue Method of Health Through Motion*. New York, New York: HarperCollins.

Fenby, J. (2008). *China's Imperial Dynasties 1600 BC - AD 1912.* Metro Books, New York: Metro Books.

Huang, K. a. R. (1987). *I Ching*. New York, New York: Workman Publishing Company.

Jingru, L., & Youqing, M. (2001). *Classical Baguazhang: Cheng Shi Baguazhang (Cheng Family Baguazhang)* (J. Crandall, Trans. II). Pinole, California: Smiling Tiger Martial Arts.

Johnson, J. J. (2000). *Barefoot Zen: The Shaolin Roots of Kung Fu and Karate*. York Beach, Maine: Samuel Weiser, Inc.

Jou, T. H. (2000). *The Tao of I Ching Way to Divination*. Scottsdale, Arizona: Tai Chi Foundation.

Jou, T. H. (2000). *The Tao of Meditation Way to Enlightenment*. Scottsdale, Arizona: Tai Chi Foundation.

Jou, T. H. (1991). *The Tao of Tai-Chi Chuan: Way to Rejuvenation*. Warwick, New York: Tai Chi Foundation.

Kennedy, B., & Guo, E. (2005). *Chinese Martial Arts Training Manuals A Historical Survey*. Berkeley, California: Blue Snake Books.

Lie, Z. (1995). *Classical Baguazhang: Yin Style Baguazhang* (J. Crandall, Trans. V). Pinole, California: Smiling Tiger Martial Arts.

Liu, D. (1990). *The Tao of Health and Longevity: Revised and Expanded Edition*. New York, New York: Marlowe & Company.

Lutang, S. (1993). *Xing Yi Quan Xue The Study of Form-Mind Boxing* (A. Liu, & D. Miller, Trans.). Pacific Grove, California:.

Lutang, S. (2002). *Classical Baguazhang: Sun Style Baguazhang (Bagua Quan Xue and Bagu Lian Xue)* (J. Crandall, Trans. XIII). Pinole, California: Smiling Tiger Martial Arts.

Lutang, S. (2003). *A Study of Taijiquan by Sun Lutang* (T. Cartmell, Trans.). Berkeley, California: North Atlantic Books.

Ming, L. Z. (1993). *Liang Zhen Pu Eight Diagram Palm* (G. Q. Huang, & V. Black, Trans.). Pacific Grove, California: High View Publications.

Mitchell, S. (1991). *Tao Te Ching A New English Version.* New York, New York: Harper Perennial.

Ni, M. P. (1995). *The Yellow Emperor's Classic of Medicine.* Boston, Massachusetts: Shambhala.

Pine, R. (1987). *The Zen Teaching of Bodhidharma.* New York, New York: North Point Press.

Ritsema, R., & Karcher, S. (1995). *I Ching The Classic Chinese Oracle of Change.* New York, New York: Barnes & Noble Books.

Smith, R. W. (2003). *Hsing-I Chinese Mind-Body Boxing.* Berkeley, California: North Atlantic Books.

Smith, R. W. (2003). *Pa-Kua Chinese Boxing for Fitness & Self-Defense.* Berkeley, California: North Atlantic Books.

Stafford, T., & Webb, M. (2005). *Mind Hacks.* 1005 Gravenstein Highway North Sebastopol, CA 95472: O'Reilly Media, Inc.

Star, J. (2001). *Tao Te Ching The Definitive Edition.* New York, New York: Penguin Group Inc.

Wilhelm, R., & Baynes, C. F. (1997). *The I Ching or Book of Changes.* Princeton, New Jersey: Princeton University Press.

Wong, E. (1997). *The Shambhala Guide To Taoism.* Boston, Massachusetts: Shambhala Publications, Inc.

IMAGES

Images of historical figures in the Foundations section of this book are from WikiPedia's public domain repository, and assumed to be in the public domain.

See http://en.wikipedia.org/wiki/Public_domain for more information.

www.ingramcontent.com/pod-product-compliance
Lightning Source LLC
Chambersburg PA
CBHW060840280326
41934CB00007B/863
* 9 7 8 0 9 8 1 9 6 7 5 2 3 *